ACLS: Rapid Reference

Ken Grauer, MD, F.A.A.F.P.

Professor, Department of Community Health and Family Medicine
Assistant Director, Family Practice Residency Program
College of Medicine, University of Florida, Gainesville
ACLS Affiliate Faculty for Florida

Dr. Grauer can be reached by:

Mail- Dr. Ken Grauer
       Family Practice Residency Program
       625 S.W. 4th Avenue
       P.O. Box 147001
       Gainesville, Florida 32614

Fax- (352) 332-9154
e-Mail- grauer@fpmg.health.ufl.edu
Home page- http://www.med.ufl.edu/chfm/people/grauer/

Daniel Cavallaro, REMT-P

Senior Medical Officer for Lifeguard Air Ambulance
President of the Center for Medical Research, Tampa, Florida
Past ACLS National Affiliate Faculty

Dan Cavallaro can be reached by:

e-Mail- danlcav@aol.com

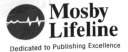
Mosby Lifeline

Dedicated to Publishing Excellence

Vice-President and Publisher: David Dusthimer
Editor-in-Chief: Rick Weimer
Manager, Business Development: Cathy Austin
Senior Assistant Editor: Kay Beard
Project Manager: Doug Bruce
Book Design: E.L. Graphics
Cover Design: Nancy McDonald

Printed in the United States of America
Composition by: E.L. Graphics
Printing/binding by: Colour Graphics Communication Group

Mosby-Year Book, Inc.
11830 Westline Industrial Drive
St. Louis, Missouri 63146

International Standard Book Number 0-8151-3831-8

97 98 99 00 01/ 9 8 7 6 5 4 3 2 1

About This New Edition of the ACLS Rapid Reference

Since publication of our 1994 ACLS Pocket Reference- *much has changed*. As a result, we have completely revised and rewritten our **ACLS Rapid Reference**. Key features included in this fruit of our labor are the following:

- Close conformance with the guidelines presented in the American Heart Association ACLS Textbook. To facilitate integration of our material with AHA Guidelines- we frequently cite *specific page numbers* in the AHA Text where relevant commentary can be found.

- Enhanced coordination with our other *new* ACLS materials. Our *Approach to the KEY Algorithms* that we present in Sections A through D of this Rapid Reference (*on pages 1-134*) consolidates the content of the initial overview chapter in our new book (**ACLS: Rapid Review and Case Scenarios**- Mosby Lifeline, 1996). It is also the synthesis of the content from the initial section in the 3rd edition of our **ACLS: Rapid Study Card Review** (Mosby Lifeline, 1996).

- *Questions to Further Understanding* that follow discussion of each of the major treatment algorithms (beginning on pages 38, 91, and 131 of this Rapid Reference). Detailed explained answers are provided to crystallize key concepts in ACLS.

- Brief general overview of pediatric resuscitation, with a detailed *user-friendly* guide to *Pediatric Drug Dosing* (pages 135-149).

- *Value Added* **ACLS Drug Table** (on pages 150-171)- to facilitate ready recall of the essentials for use of the 20 most important drugs in ACLS.

- Ever increased *USER-Friendliness* of this Rapid Reference- by inclusion of our *Table of Contents* and *Quick-Find Index* on the inside front and back covers. Rapid retrieval of *whatever* information you are seeking is an instant reality.

- An opportunity for direct contact with *YOU*- our readers. We *welcome* your feedback, questions, and concerns! We have therefore included our mailing address, fax number, and e-mail address (on the *Title Page* of this Rapid Reference) to facilitate receiving your comments.

We sincerely hope this Rapid Reference is of interest (and is helpful) to you. It was written with *YOU* (our readers) in mind.

Ken Grauer, MD
Dan Cavallaro, REMT-P

For Those Who Want to Know More...

(Other related material written by these authors)

- Grauer K, Cavallaro D: **ACLS: Rapid Review and Case Scenarios**- 4th Edition (Mosby Lifeline- 1996) - Book code 28155- $ 19.95

- Grauer K, Cavallaro D: **ACLS: Rapid Study Card Review**- 3rd Edition (Mosby Lifeline- 1997) - Book code 28177- $ 27.95

- Grauer K, Cavallaro D: **Arrhythmia Interpretation: ACLS Preparation & Clinical Approach** (Mosby Lifeline- *Expected publication in January, 1997*) Book code 28156 $ 23.95

- Grauer K: **A Practical Guide to ECG Interpretation** (Mosby-Year Book- 1992) Book code 02159- $ 32.95

Call 1-800 MOSBY-N-U

(1-800-667-2968)

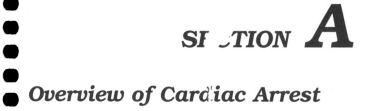

Overview of Cardiac Arrest

The goal of this ACLS Rapid Reference is to consolidate information from our other ACLS materials into a user-friendly format that can easily be applied *at the bedside-* for help in management of the patient in cardiac arrest (or with impending arrest). This work can either be used independently- or as a study guide in conjunction with any of our other ACLS materials.

Grading of AHA Recommendations

Application of scientific evidence to the *nearly-impossible-to-control-for* clinical situation of cardiopulmonary arrest poses a true dilemma. A **Grading System** for classifying **Therapeutic Interventions** in ACLS has been developed by a panel of experts in an attempt to integrate in the most objective manner possible the relative strength of *available* supporting evidence for recommendations put forth in the AHA Guidelines. Grading according to this classification is as follows (AHA Text- Pg 1-10):

- **Class I**- a therapetuic option that is *usually indicated,* always acceptable- and considered useful and effective.

- **Class II**- a therapeutic option that is *acceptable*, is of uncertain efficacy- and may be controversial.

  - **Class IIa**- a therapeutic option for which the weight of evidence is *in favor* of its usefulness and efficacy.

  - **Class IIb**- a therapeutic option that is *not* well established by evidence, but may be helpful (and probably is *not* harmful).

- **Class III**- a therapeutic option that is inappropriate, is without scientific supporting data- and may be harmful.

The grading classification may be *summarized* as follows:

> ■ **Class I**- *definitely* helpful!
>
>   ■ **Class IIa**- *probably* helpful.
>
>   ■ **Class IIb**- *possibly* helpful.
>
>   ■ **Class III**- *not* indicated.
>   (*and possibly harmful*)

The reason for developing a grading system is simple: a need existed for more objective (and more scientific) discrimination between the various treatment options available.   Clinicians faced with sifting through an extensive imperfect literature needed guidance.

As helpful as having graded recommendations is, the clinician is still left with a problem: *What to do at the bedside (or on the scene)- when the patient is **coding** and universally accepted beneficial (i.e., Class I) interventions are simply **not** working?* In such situations- ***judgement is needed** on the part of the emergency care provider* to determine the most suitable management approach for the particular clinical situation at hand.

> **Bottom Line**- Application of Class I recommendations is clearly preferable whenever this is possible. Interventions graded as Class III are to be avoided. In between- *judgement is needed.*

Examples of Grading ACLS Interventions

Insight into the ***Grading System*** for ACLS interventions is probably best provided by citing clinical examples for the more commonly used therapies in each class.

■ Examples of ***Class I*** (i.e., *definitely* helpful) interventions:

-   **S**tandard-**D**ose **E**pinephrine (***SDE***) = 1 mg IV every 3-5 minutes in the treatment of V Fib.
- ***"Stacked"* Defibrillations**- for persistent V Fib (especially when administration of medication is delayed).
- ***Sodium Bicarbonate***- *IF* (and *only* if) the patient has known *preexisting* hyperkalemia (*See Class III recommendations below.*)

- **Lidocaine** and/or **Procainamide**- for treatment of *wide-complex* tachycardia of *uncertain* etiology.
- **Magnesium Sulfate**- for cardiac arrest/Acute MI when there is known (or suspected) magnesium deficiency; and/or for suppression of *Torsade de Pointes*.

■ Examples of **Class IIa** (i.e., *probably* helpful) interventions:

- **Antifibrillatory Agents** (i.e., **Lidocaine- Bretylium**)- for persistent V Fib. (In reality, the efficacy of these drugs in the latter stages of cardiopulmonary resuscitation is unknown).
- **Adenosine**- for treatment of a *wide-complex* tachycardia of *unknown* etiology (although this drug is unlikely to be helpful if the rhythm turns out to be VT).
- **Trans**Cutaneous **P**acing **(TCP)**- is a Class IIa recommenda-tion for drug resistant bradycardia when there is an escape rhythm.

> **Note**- Pacing is a **Class I** recommendation for hemodynamically compromising bradycardias- *but* it is **Class IIb** for asystole (because TCP is *unlikely* to save such patients- unless started very *early* in the code).

■ Examples of **Class IIb** (i.e., *possibly* helpful) interventions:

- Use of *higher doses* of Epinephrine (i.e., **HDE**) during resuscitation in cases when an initial 1 mg IV dose (i.e., SDE) does not work.
- Routine use of less well studied antifibrillatory agents (i.e., **Magnesium- Procainamide**) for persistent V Fib.

> **Note**- Use of **Magnesium** becomes a **Class IIa** recommendation in the treatment of cardiac arrest for patients with low (or suspected low) serum Magnesium levels.

- **Trans**Cutaneous **P**acing **(TCP)**- for asystole (with the *KEY* to success being to institute pacing as soon as possible).
- **Atropine**- for asystole or severe AV block.

- Examples of **Class III** (i.e., *not* indicated and *possibly* harm-ful) interventions:
  - **Verapamil/Diltiazem**- for treatment of a *wide-complex* tachycardia of *unknown* etiology.
  - **Sodium Bicarbonate**- has a *variable* status (i.e., depending on the clinical situation!). It is designated as:
    - **Class I**- if the patient has *preexisting* hyperkalemia.
    - **Class IIa**- if the patient has known (or suspected) preexisting bicarbonate-responsive metabolic acidosis- or to alkalinize serum in severe tricyclic overdose.
    - **Class IIb**- for *intubated* patients in prolonged cardiac arrest- and/or after return of a pulse following prolonged arrest.
    - **Class III**- for patients with *hypoxic* lactic acidosis (as is likely to occur in *nonintubated* patients with prolonged cardiopulmonary arrest)- for whom *improved ventilation* (*and not Bicarb!*) is the treatment of choice!

The Universal Algorithm for Adult ECC (Emergency Cardiac Care)

AHA Guidelines advise regular use of the **Universal Algorithm** for the *initial* approach to adult *ECC* (*Emergency Cardiac Care*). A decided advantage of this approach is that its steps are applicable to virtually *any* emergency situation (Figure 1A-1).

> **Note**- The steps and actions encompassed in the **Universal Algorithm** are virtually *identical* to those that comprise the **Primary** and **Secondary Surveys** used in ECC. AHA Guidelines allow for use of *whichever* approach "works best for the learner" (AHA Text- Pg 1-11).

Specific points to keep in mind regarding use of the *Universal Algorithm* include the following:

- Classification of the patient (and the initial approach to management) is determined by the answers to three basic questions:

  <u>Question #1</u>- Is the patient ***responsive*** ?

  <u>Question #2</u>- Is the patient ***breathing*** ?

  <u>Question #3</u>- Is there a ***pulse*** ?

- Note that calling for help assumes *high priority* in the algorithm. Except for a few *special* situations (*see below*)- the ***Call for Help*** should be made *as soon as* the rescuer determines that the victim is unresponsive.

- <u>If the patient is *NOT* responsive, *NOT* breathing, and there is *NO* pulse</u>- then by definition, the patient is in ***full* cardiac arrest**. Carefully roll the patient over (if they are not already on their back)- and *begin* **CPR**. Specifics of subsequent management depend on the *mechanism* of the arrest. The three major mechanisms of cardiac arrest are **V Fib/Pulseless VT** (the most common mechanism)- **PEA** or **P**ulseless **E**lectrical **A**ctivity (when electrical activity in the form of an ECG rhythm is present but the patient is pulseless)- and ***asystole*** (when there is *no* electrical activity and *no* pulse). Management of these conditions is discussed in detail in Sections 1B, 1C, and 1D of this Rapid Reference.

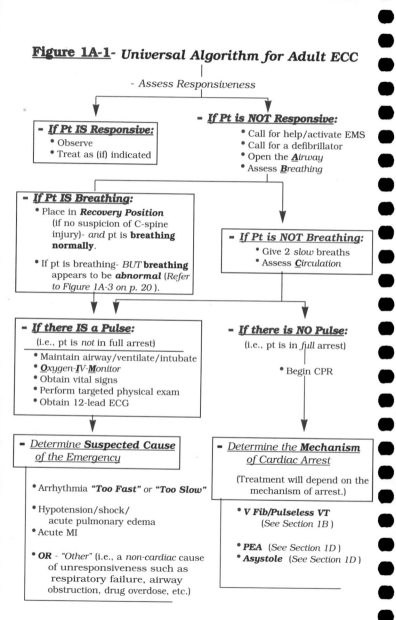

Figure 1A-1- *Universal Algorithm for Adult ECC*

- *Assess Responsiveness*

- *If Pt IS Responsive:*
- Observe
- Treat as (if) indicated

- *If Pt is NOT Responsive:*
- Call for help/activate EMS
- Call for a defibrillator
- Open the **A**irway
- Assess **B**reathing

- *If Pt IS Breathing:*
- Place in **Recovery Position** (if no suspicion of C-spine injury)- *and* pt is **breathing normally**.
- If pt is breathing- BUT **breathing** appears to be **abnormal** (*Refer to Figure 1A-3 on p. 20*).

- *If Pt is NOT Breathing:*
- Give 2 *slow* breaths
- Assess **C**irculation

- *If there IS a Pulse:*
(i.e., pt is *not* in full arrest)
- Maintain airway/ventilate/intubate
- **O**xygen-**I**V-**M**onitor
- Obtain vital signs
- Perform targeted physical exam
- Obtain 12-lead ECG

- *If there is NO Pulse:*
(i.e., pt is in *full* arrest)
- Begin CPR

- Determine *Suspected Cause* of the Emergency

- Arrhythmia ***"Too Fast"*** or ***"Too Slow"***
- Hypotension/shock/ acute pulmonary edema
- Acute MI
- **OR** - *"Other"* (i.e., a *non-cardiac* cause of unresponsiveness such as respiratory failure, airway obstruction, drug overdose, etc.)

- Determine the *Mechanism* of Cardiac Arrest

(Treatment will depend on the mechanism of arrest.)

- **V Fib/Pulseless VT** (*See Section 1B*)
- **PEA** (*See Section 1D*)
- **Asystole** (*See Section 1D*)

■ If the patient is <u>*unresponsive*- but *IS* breathing</u>- then the patient is *not* in full arrest (i.e., a pulse *will* be present). The patient's airway should be maintained while the rescuer assesses the efficacy of breathing:

    - <u>If breathing appears to be normal</u>- the patient should be placed in the **recovery position** (provided that there is *no suspicion* of C-spine injury- *See Page 8*).

    - <u>If breathing appears to be *abnormal*</u>- the rescuer should *reposition* the airway and reassess the situation. The objectives of management at this point are to rule out any component of airway obstruction- and take measures to ensure that ventilation and oxygenation are both adequate.

> **KEY**- If a pulse *is* present- then by definition, the patient is *not* in full arrest. In this situation, one of three types of respiratory patterns may be present:
>   i) normal breathing
>   ii) abnormal breathing
>   iii) no breathing at all.

■ <u>For the patient who is *not* in full arrest</u>- initial efforts are aimed at ensuring that ventilation and oxygenation are both adequate. After accomplishing this, attention is directed at determining the predominant/underlying *cause* of the cardiopulmonary emergency.

    A *combination* of factors is often responsible for the patient's condition. For example, acute myocardial infarction may precipitate cardiogenic shock if the infarct is large- *resulting in* hypotension, pulmonary edema, and ventricular tachyarrhythmias. Bradycardia might also be seen if an extensive infarction affects the conduction system. Superimposed development of severe 2° or 3° AV block would certainly aggravate the patient's already compromised hemodynamic condition. As might be imagined, treatment depends on identifying the primary cause(s) of hemodynamic decompensation- and intervening appropriately.

> ***Note*-** A *non-cardiac* cause may also be responsible for the patient's condition. Important **non-cardiac causes** of *unresponsiveness* to consider include respiratory failure, complete airway obstruction, drug overdose, CNS catastrophe (such as a stroke or intracerebral hemorrhage), severe electrolyte abnormality, post-ictal state- and others.

- Finally- we draw attention to a *series* of **Supportive Actions** that should be initiated near the beginning of most of the AHA algorithms for treatment. These actions include:
    - Maintenance of the airway/ventilation/intubation.
    - **O**xygen-**I**V-**M**onitor (which AHA Guidelines suggest grouping as a *single* "word" to facilitate rapid implementation (AHA Text- Pg 1-27). Specifically, use of this action entails provision of supplemental **O**xygen- establishment of **I**V access- and attachment of **M**onitoring leads to the patient.
    - Obtaining vital signs (as appropriate).
    - Performance of a *targeted* physical exam.
    - Obtaining a 12-lead ECG (as soon as this becomes clinically feasible).

The Recovery Position

As noted in the *Universal Algorithm* (Figure 1A-1)- if the patient is unresponsive but breathing normally, use of the **recovery position** is advised (Figure 1A-2).

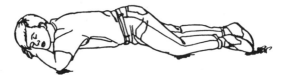

Figure 1A-2: The Recovery Position

Placement of the victim into the recovery position should *not* be attempted if there is *any* suspicion of C-spine injury. However, in the absence of this concern- moving the patient into this position minimizes the chance of developing airway obstruction that could otherwise be precipitated in the supine position (by the tongue falling back to occlude the airway). Use of the recovery position also minimizes the chance of aspiration by facilitating spontaneous drainage of the victim's secretions.

Special Situations: The *Lone* Rescuer

A dilemma arises when a trained health care provider finds himself/herself *alone* on the scene of a cardiopulmonary arrest- and *no one* is able to hear the call for help. The problem confronting the **lone rescuer** is what to do next:

    i) *Stay with the victim* (and perform 1-rescuer CPR)?

        or

    ii) *Leave the victim* (to try to find help)?

In the past, AHA Guidelines called for the *single* rescuer to remain with the victim and perform 1-person CPR for an initial *one minute* prior to activating the EMS system. Despite its intuitive appeal, in practice this recommendation frequently led to significant delays in defibrillation. Awareness of time passage at the scene of an actual arrest is often imprecise- and if left to their own, trained *single* rescuers tend to perform CPR for much *longer* than the recommended "minute" before calling EMS. Practically speaking, the overwhelming majority of adults with sudden non-traumatic out-of-hospital cardiac arrest who are *potentially salvageable* will be in V Fib by the time EMS personnel arrive on the scene. For many of these patients, delay for the minute (or more) that it takes to access the EMS system could spell the difference between neurologically intact survival and a far less optimal outcome.

On the other hand, concern about recommending that the rescuer *always* leave the victim to immediately access EMS is valid. This is because *some* adults (who have either pure *respiratory* arrest or a completely *obstructed airway*) may be *inappropriately* treated by delaying full assessment of the victim and initial ventilatory support for the time that it takes to activate the EMS system. If the duration of this delay is at all prolonged (as it is likely to be if the *lone* rescuer is isolated from a phone or other access modality)- failure to *immediately* initiate ventilatory assistance could result in failure to save the patient (or in resuscitation with a less than optimal neurologic outcome). Clearly then- there *are* situations in which ensuring a patent airway and initiating rescue breathing assume *higher priority* than leaving the victim to immediately access EMS.

> **Bottom Line**- Judgement is needed (and *individualized* decision making is advised) on the part of the single *trained* rescuer for deciding what to do *first* at the scene of an apparent cardiopulmonary arrest (AHA Text- Pg 1-5).

Specific points to keep in mind regarding the approach we suggest for the **lone** rescuer are listed below. Note that the approach recommended *differs* for the trained rescuer than for the layperson rescuer.

- For the <u>untrained</u> **Lay Rescuer**:

  - AHA Guidelines emphasize the need for a clear and *simple* message (in order to encourage action- yet minimize the chance of confusion). Lay individuals are easily intimidated by (and have difficulty remembering) complex decision analysis protocols- especially when called upon to render assistance in a life or death situation in which the victim may be a loved one. AHA Guidelines have therefore *simplified* the message to the single lay rescuer to- **"Phone FIRST"** - as soon as they encounter an unresponsive victim.

- For the <u>trained</u> **Professional Rescuer** (who is *able to appreciate* the subtleties involved):

  - If *pure* **respiratory arrest** is suspected (i.e., from airway obstruction, drowning, drug overdose, etc.)- **STAY** *at the scene* with the victim. *Immediately* initiate rescue breathing, since this action could be *lifesaving* in this situation.

  - Application of a Heimlich maneuver (i.e., abdominal thrusts)- *is* appropriate as an *initial* measure for the victim who is *known* (or strongly suspected) to have foreign-body airway obstruction. The most common clinical example of this situation involves the sudden collapse of a healthy adult in a restaurant setting- especially when the victim is last seen abruptly getting up from the table and rushing toward the bathroom.

- If *cardiac* **arrest** is suspected as the cause of collapse, and help is "nearby" (i.e., *within* 1-2 minutes away)- *LEAVE the victim and run to get help.* Call EMS. Then *return* to the victim *as soon as you can* and initiate CPR until the EMS unit arrives on the scene.

- Remember that the overwhelming majority of *adult* victims of sudden death die from *cardiac* arrest (and *not* from respiratory arrest). Defibrillation at the earliest possible moment holds the *KEY* for improving survival. Placing the call to activate the EMS system *immediately* after discovering the victim is the best way to expedite the process.

- If *doubt* exists as to the cause of an arrest- always assume a *cardiac* etiology and act accordingly (i.e., *call EMS first!*). Then *return* to the victim and perform CPR until the EMS unit arrives on the scene. Take comfort in the fact that even trained rescuers often have great difficulty and may be *unable* to distinguish between primary cardiac arrest, and collapse that is secondary to airway or breathing problems.

- Admittedly, if you are **all alone** at the scene when the victim collapses, and **help is *not* nearby**- *"You face some tough decisions"* (AHA Text- Pg 1-6). AHA Guidelines cite the example of sudden collapse of a jogging partner on an isolated trail *remote* from any assistance or phone contact. Sudden development of pulselessness in a jogger is almost certain indication of V Fib or pulseless VT. Realistically speaking, if help is far away (i.e., *more* than 5-10 minutes away)- the chance of accessing such help *in time* to save a collapsed victim in V Fib is practically nil. In this situation AHA Guidelines state that "common sense suggests the trained health care professional will ensure an open airway, attempt several precordial thumps, and continue CPR for at least 10 to 15 minutes" (AHA Text- Pg 1-6). Practically speaking- *not much else can be done* when you are all alone without access to a defibrillator.

- The approach recommended for the lone rescuer is different if the victim is an **infant** or **child**. In this situation, rapid assessment to rule out respiratory obstruction, and action to ensure adequate ventilation should be done *first* (i.e., *before* accessing EMS)- because of the much greater likelihood that an airway problem will be the primary cause of collapse or distress. AHA Guidelines advise the lone rescuer to provide an ***initial* one minute of rescue support** *before* seeking to access EMS personnel (AHA Text- Pg 16-7).

Use of Barrier Devices: *Practical Considerations*

Because of concern about the possibility of disease transmission, health care providers may be reluctant to initiate CPR on an unknown victim of cardiopulmonary arrest. In acknowledgement of this potential risk, we emphasize the following specific points:

■ Statistically, out-of-hospital cardiac arrest is most likely to occur in the home. As a result- *layperson* CPR will most often be administered by an individual who is either related to and/or aware of the victim's health status. In such cases, there is usually little reluctance to perform CPR (including mouth-to-mouth ventilation)- provided that the rescuer is capable of doing so.

In contrast, health care providers who encounter an *out-of-hospital* situation in which they are called on to administer CPR will usually *not* know the victim- and therefore *not* be aware of the victim's health status. Not knowing this information is a major reason why health care providers may choose not to perform mouth-to-mouth rescue breathing in this situation.

- There clearly *is* potential opportunity for saliva exchange to occur between victim and rescuer during mouth-to-mouth resuscitation. However, the *actual* risk of transmitting either hepatitis B virus or HIV infection as a *direct* result of performing CPR appears to be exceedingly small. This risk is even less if the skin around the lips and within the oral mucosa of the rescuer is intact.

- Administration of mouth-to-mouth rescue breathing may entail a somewhat greater risk of disease transmission to the rescuer if the recipient is infected with herpes simplex, Neisseria meningitidis, tuberculosis, and/or certain other types of pulmonary infections. Fortunately, even in these cases- the *overall* risk of disease transmission is probably still quite small.

- Increased availability and use of **barrier** **methods** (i.e., latex gloves, face masks or face shields, bag-valve devices, etc.) should help to *minimize* the risk of disease transmission to the rescuer. Ready availability of these devices will hopefully also reduce the reluctance of health care providers to perform rescue breathing.

- Be aware of the clinical reality that if you encounter a victim of cardiopulmonary arrest *outside* of a hospital (or other medical setting) and *YOU* do not perform CPR- *the chances are good that no one else will.* In this situation the patient will probably die. If the cause of the arrest is *purely* respiratory in nature (as it is likely to be with victims of drowning or drug overdose)- prompt adminstration of rescue breathing could be a potentially *lifesaving* intervention . . .

- On the other hand, if a patient arrests *within* a hospital (or other medical setting) and you *know* help (and a *barrier* respiratory device) is on the way- it is probably reasonable to wait a few moments for such help to arrive. VT/V Fib is by far the most common cause of cardiopulmonary arrest in this setting- for which *defibrillation* is the treatment of choice. Putting off management of the airway for a few moments (although less than ideal) will probably *not* adversely affect outcome in most instances.

- Knowledge that nothing in the patient's history *even remotely* suggests that he/she might be HIV positive or have hepatitis B, herpes, active tuberculosis, or meningococcal meningitis- is information that *might* affect your decision of whether to administer mouth-to-mouth rescue breathing.

- If you decide *NOT* to administer rescue breathing- **_Remember_** *that performing a few cycles of external chest compressions is BETTER than doing nothing.* A primary cardiac arrest victim usually still has a certain amount of oxygenated blood in his or her system- and performance of chest compressions (at least for a *few* cycles) may help to circulate some of this blood.

- Greater **anticipation** (on the part of health care providers) should help to facilitate more widespread and appropriate use of respiratory barrier devices. For example, hospital staff could work to identify which acutely ill patients are at greatest risk of developing respiratory or cardiac arrest. They could then make it a point to have barrier devices routinely available at the bedside of these high risk patients.

  An even more fundamental **anticipatory issue** to address in hospitalized patients (*before* the arrest occurs!) is the question of whether cardiopulmonary resuscitation is even indicated or desired at all . . . . .

We Suggest- Consider setting aside a moment *NOW* for **self-reflection** on your part- as to how **YOU** feel it will be most appropriate to act in the event you are one day confronted with the problematic issue of whether to administer mouth-to-mouth resuscitation to a nonbreathing victim of cardiopulmonary arrest. A moment of anticipatory reflection *at THIS time* may be *invaluable* for facilitating the decision-making process (as well as *expediting* your actions) in the event that you do encounter this situation at some time in the future (*which you probably will!*). You might also consider the purchase of an inexpensive, portable barrier device (from your neighborhood pharmacy) to either keep in your car or on your person- *just in case . . . .*

How to Optimize CPR

Good technical performance of CPR *is* important. Having stated this, we feel it important to emphasize the clinical reality that by itself- performance of even perfect CPR will *not* prevent V Fib from deteriorating to asystole. What prompt initiation of CPR may do is *delay* deterioration of the rhythm- and in so doing *preserve viability* (i.e., responsiveness to defibrillation) for at least a short period of time (of perhaps 1-2 minutes). Prolonging the period of potential viability could prove to be *lifesaving* if defibrillation can then be accomplished in a timely manner.

Despite much research in this area, the actual mechanism for explaining how CPR works is *not* yet completely clear. Nevertheless, what *does* seem clear is that the *efficacy* of CPR can be enhanced by attention to several key parameters. These include:

- **Ventilating *slowly* and effectively**. Ventilations should be delivered over an inspiratory time of *at least* 1.0 (and preferably closer to 2.0) seconds per breath. In addition to ventilating slowly, the rescuer should ensure that the chest actually rises with each breath delivered. The sensation of air as it enters and expands the lungs should be *felt* by the rescuer with each respiration. If this does not occur- then the airway is *not* completely patent. This may either be due to inadequate airway control (which should resolve, or at least improve with *repositioning* of the victim)- or to a mechanical cause (such as a foreign body).

    As already emphasized, the importance of ventilating *slowly* is that this intervention improves the efficiency of rescue breathing by allowing adequate time for chest expansion. An additional reason for slowing the rate of ventilation in the *nonintubated* patient is that doing so reduces the risk of producing gastric distention (with resultant regurgitation/aspiration)- because it lessens the chance that esophageal opening pressure will be exceeded during any given rescue breath.

- **Compressing with *adequate* (but *not* excessive) force**. One should *not* use 'rib-breaking' force- but enough force to *adequately* depress the sternum. Failure to do so may significantly reduce the impetus for blood flow during CPR. AHA Guidelines recommend depressing the chest by 1.5-2.0 inches with each compression in the adult victim.

> **_KEY_**- It should be emphasized that performance of CPR is *not* benign. In addition to the almost universal subjective complaint of "sore chest" reported by CPR survivors- more serious complications (i.e., pneumothorax, pericardial tamponade, flail chest) occur in a significant percentage of patients. Although some of these injuries are clearly unavoidable- others (i.e., fractures of the *lateral* portion of a rib, or fractures of the *lower* ribs) could possibly have been prevented if CPR technique was more proficient (using correct hand placement over the lower half of the sternum, avoiding finger contact on the lateral chest wall when compressing, not being overzealous with application of force, etc.)

- **Compressing at the *higher end* of the rate range**. The recommended range for adults is to compress at a rate of between **80-100/minute**- and *not* at a rate of 1 per second as is still all too commonly done! Cardiac output during CPR is directly related to the *duration* of chest compression. As the rate of compression increases, the relative *percentage* of time that comprises the compression phase of CPR becomes proportionately greater (compared to the time that comprises relaxation). In addition, rescuers tend to apply greater *force* with each compression when working at a faster rate (*high-impulse CPR*). Thus the end result of increasing the recommended rate for chest compressions is improved efficiency of CPR because the faster rate *proportionately* lengthens the period of compression duration as it increases the *force* applied with each compression. Aiming for the *upper end* of the rate range for compressions (i.e., compressing as close to a rate of 100/minute as possible- especially during the early minutes of the resuscitation effort) may be the most effective noninvasive way to optimize blood flow during CPR.

- **Considering use of _Epinephrine_ at the _earliest_ opportunity**. Without CPR, blood will _not_ flow in the arrested heart. With properly performed two-rescuer CPR- cardiac output may approach up to 25% of normal values. However, despite this beneficial effect, the unfortunate clinical reality is that by itself- CPR is _not_ an effective way to achieve adequate blood flow to the organs that count (i.e., to the heart and the brain). Practically speaking, unless vasoconstrictor medication such as Epinephrine is used, blood flow to these essential organs is virtually nil in the arrested heart (even when excellent quality CPR is being performed!). Use of Epinephrine is therefore recommended at an _early_ point in the treatment of cardiac arrest- and the drug should be repeated _often_ (i.e., at 3 to 5 minute intervals) if the patient fails to respond.

- **_Monitoring the process_**. All too often, cardiopulmonary resuscitation at the bedside of a hospitalized patient becomes an overcrowded event. An important function that extra health care providers may serve at the bedside is to _monitor_ the quality of CPR being performed, and constructively provide _ongoing_ feedback to rescuers on parameters of CPR that they may not be aware of. For example- when left to their own, emergency care providers tend to slow down the rate of external chest compression as the code progresses. Furthermore, many health care providers are completely _unaware_ of the actual rate at which they are compressing.

We Suggest- _Prove this to yourself._ The next time you are an "extra" person at the scene of a cardiopulmonary arrest- _stand back_ for a moment, and _monitor_ the overall process. _Count the compression rate._ Observe other aspects of CPR performance (i.e., whether a bed board is used, compression technique, efficacy of ventilation, etc.). Given the importance of optimizing blood flow during CPR- your **ongoing feedback** could make a difference in the ultimate outcome of the code.

Consideration might be given to the use of some *objective* method for timing (and pacing the rate of) cardiac compressions. This may be done with a **metronome** (as is used to keep time in music) or an *audiorecording*. Use of an audio-prompted, rate-directing signal in this manner is a simple, practical way to ensure *awareness* of the correct rate of compressions. This not only facilitates the ability of rescuers to *maintain* the rate of compressions within the correct range *throughout* the resuscitation effort- but as noted above, it may also lead to significant improvement in the efficacy of compressions.

Algorithm for Management of the Adult Airway

To help conceptualize our approach to the patient with respiratory difficulty, we have developed an Algorithm for *Management of the Adult Airway* (Figure 1A-3). The management sequence begins with the rescuer *simultaneously* assessing ventilation and the level of consciousness (**1**).

Note- Many definitions exist for the terms conscious, semiconscious, and unconscious. For the purpose of determining optimal management of the airway, we have defined these terms in the following manner:

- **Conscious** - a patient who is alert, awake, and responding appropriately.

- **Semiconscious** - a less alert patient who may not be awake and only responds to verbal or painful stimuli. The gag reflex may still be intact.

- **Unconscious** - a patient who cannot be aroused and does not respond to either verbal or painful stimuli. The gag reflex is absent.

If a patient is conscious or semiconscious and spontaneously breathing in a *normal* manner- all that may be needed is supplemental oxygen (**1-2-4**). The rescuer should then evaluate the adequacy of oxygenation (**5**). This may be done by physical

Figure 1A-3- *Algorithm for Management of the Adult Airway*

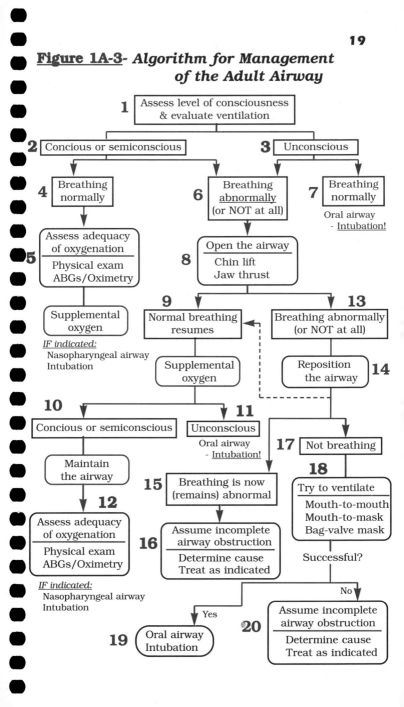

examination, oximetry, and/or by arterial blood gas sampling (if indicated). If this evaluation suggests that oxygenation is inadequate- more definitive management of the airway (either by insertion of a nasopharyngeal airway or endotracheal intubation) is needed.

> **Note**- Unconscious patients (even if they appear to be breathing normally)- require definitive airway management with endotracheal intubation (**1-3-7**).

For patients who are breathing *abnormally* (and for those who are *not* breathing at all)- appropriate management of the airway is the same *regardless* of the state of consciousness (**1-2-6**) or (**1-3-6**). In either case, the airway should be manually opened by either the chin-lift or jaw-thrust maneuver (**8**). If this results in resumption of normal breathing (**9**)- supplemental oxygen should be administered. For the unconscious patient, definitive airway management with endotracheal intubation is again the treatment of choice (**6-8-9-11**). On the other hand, if the patient is conscious or semiconscious (**10**)- less definitive therapy may be needed. Manually maintain the airway. Further management will then hinge on assessment of the adequacy of oxygenation (**6-8-9-10-12**).

If after initially opening the airway, the patient continues to breathe *abnormally* (or is still *not* breathing at all)- the rescuer should *reposition* the airway (**6-8-13-14**). If this results in resumption of normal breathing, management should follow the course described above (**8-9-10-12**) or (**8-9-11**). On the other hand, if breathing is still *abnormal* after repositioning the airway (**15**)- the rescuer should assume incomplete airway obstruction is present, and treat accordingly (**6-8-13-14-15-16**).

If the patient remains in respiratory arrest even after repositioning the airway- an attempt should be made to ventilate the patient (**14-17-18**). If successful, definitive airway management with endotracheal intubation should be performed (**19**). If unsuccessful, the rescuer should assume complete airway obstruction, and treat accordingly (**20**).

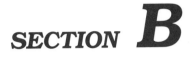

V Fib/Pulseless VT

By far, the most common precipitating mechanism of car-diopulmonary arrest in adults is V Fib/Pulseless VT. Depending on the setting of the arrest (i.e., *inside* or *outside* of the hospital)-and depending on what criteria are used to identify the *precipi-tating mechanism* (i.e., the initial rhythm documented by hospi-tal or EMS personnel)- **V Fib** or **Pulseless VT** may be found on arrival at the scene in up to 80% of nontraumatic cardiac arrests in adults.

Treatment Algorithm: *Initial Actions*

In <u>Figure 1B-1</u> we illustrate the *initial* approach recom-mended by AHA Guidelines for the patient who is found in **V Fib/Pulseless VT**. Note that the algorithm assumes **the rhythm is real** (i.e., that the patient is *truly* pulseless- and that the ECG recording is *not* the result of artifact).

- Although not shown in Figure 1B-1- resuscitative efforts routinely begin with the **Universal Algorithm** (<u>Figure 1A-1</u>- on page 6)- in which *responsiveness* of the victim is first assessed and the **ABC**s (of **A**irway/**B**reathing/**C**irculation) are attended to.

- We emphasize that the single *most* important interven-tion in adult emergency cardiac care (*by far!*) is defibrillation. Regardless of the setting in which car-diac arrest occurs (i.e., *home- community-* or in the *hospital*)- successful adult resuscitation depends most often on *early* defibrillation.

> **_KEY_**- The *sooner* a patient in V Fib/pulseless VT is defibrillated- the *better* the chance for long-term survival.

- **Initial Series of Countershocks**- AHA recommendations for energy level selections to use for the initial
series of countershocks are as follows (AHA Text- Pg
1-15):

  - **1st Shock**- 200 joules
  - **2nd Shock**- 200-300 joules
  - **3rd Shock**- 360 joules

  We favor routine use of the higher energy level
  (300 joules) for the 2nd countershock attempt-
  because this provides for a "more predictable
  increase in current" (AHA Text- Pg 4-6).

- AHA Guidelines recommend delivery of countershocks in
"stacked" sequence (i.e., *one right after another*) for
the *initial* defibrillation series. Rescuers should *not*
pause for a pulse check between countershock
attempts. Minimizing the time between shock
attempts in this manner helps to ensure rapid delivery of the initial defibrillation series. It also reduces
TTR (*TransThoracic Resistance*) of the victim's chest
wall- and therefore allows a greater amount of *current*
to pass through the victim's heart with the 2nd
shock.

- Even *after* delivery of the first three shocks- AHA
Guidelines now allow for *continued* delivery of shock
attempts in *stacked* sequence. Continued use of
stacked shocks in "sets" of three (with energies from
200-360 joules) might be especially appropriate for
treatment of patients with persistent V Fib when
administration of medication is delayed (AHA Text-
Pg 1-18).

- **Pulse checks**- are *no longer recommended* in between
shocks of a stacked series- provided that rescuers
can be *confident* that the monitor is correctly hooked
up, and that the rhythm being displayed is *truly* V Fib
(AHA Text- Pg 1-15). Instead, all efforts are best
directed at confirming V Fib- and then working to
deliver *successive* shocks in a series *as rapidly as
possible.*

Figure 1B-1- *Treatment Algorithm for V Fib/Pulseless VT* (Initial Approach)

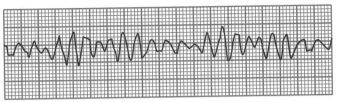

Initial Actions:

- ABCs/Perform CPR until defibrillator attached/Confirm V Fib.
  - ■ **Shock** (up to **3 times** in *stacked* sequence- *if/as needed*) for persistent V Fib/Pulseless VT: *(p. 22)*

    - Use energy levels of **200j**- **200-300j**- and then **360 joules**.

    > ***NOTE-*** *NO pulse check is needed between shocks that are given in stacked sequence!*

If V Fib/Pulseless VT persists:

- Continue CPR/Intubate/Establish IV access.
  - ■ **Epinephrine:** *(p. 24)*
    - Use an **SDE** dose (i.e., **1.0 mg** by IV bolus) initially.
    - May *either* repeat SDE (every 3-5 minutes- if/as needed)-
      - or *increase* the dose (i.e., to **HDE**) if there has been no response, choosing between several HDE regimens:

    i) *"Intermediate"* dose Epinephrine = **2-5 mg** IV boluses
      - *OR* -
        ii) *Escalating* **1- 3- 5 mg** IV boluses
          - *OR* -
            iii) Dosing at **0.1 mg/kg** as an IV bolus.

  - ■ **Shock** (within 30-60 seconds after 1st Epinephrine dose):
    - Use *either* **360j** as a *single* shock- *or* may again shock in *stacked sequence* (with another series of 3 successive shocks at 200-360j).

    > ***NOTE-*** *Use of stacked shocks would be especially appropriate at this time-* ***IF*** *administration of medication is delayed.*

If V Fib/Pulseless VT Persists- _Use of Epinephrine_

If V Fib persists after the 3rd countershock attempt, other measures should be tried. These include resumption of CPR- attempting to _intubate_ the patient and establish _IV access_- and hooking the patient up to a monitor. _A trial of medications is now in order._

- **_Epinephrine_** is the drug of first choice for treatment of cardiac arrest. The most important effect of this drug in the arrested heart results from its vasoconstrictor (alpha-adrenergic) action- which serves to enhance the gradient for blood flow to the heart and brain.

- Use **S**tandard-**D**ose **E**pinephrine **(SDE)** first- giving **1.0 mg** of drug (or 10 ml of a 1:10,000 soln.) by **IV bolus**. Because the effect of an IV bolus of Epinephrine peaks in about 2-3 minutes- the drug should probably be repeated _at least_ every 3-5 minutes for as long as the patient remains in cardiac arrest.

- AHA Guidelines allow for _flexibility_ in Epinephrine dosing if the patient fails to respond to the initial SDE dose (AHA Text- Pg 1-16). One may _either_ repeat the 1 mg SDE dose in 3-5 minutes (and continue thereafter as needed with 1 mg doses)- **or** _choose between several_ **H**igh-**D**ose **alternative** _regimens._ These include:

i) Administration of **2-5 mg** IV boluses (which AHA Guidelines describe as _"intermediate"_ dose Epinephrine)

_- OR -_

ii) _Escalating_ **1- 3- 5 mg** IV boluses

_- OR -_

iii) Dosing at **0.1 mg/kg** as an IV bolus.

> **Note**- Epinephrine may also be given by the **ET route** if IV access is unavailable. A higher dose is needed than by the IV route. AHA Guidelines advise using 2-2.5 times the recommended IV dose (i.e, **2-2.5 mg** of 1:10,000 soln)- instilling this amount of drug down the ET tube- and following this with several forceful insufflations of the Ambu bag.

- If V Fib persists following Epinephrine- another (i.e., **4th**) **shock** should be given in an attempt to convert the patient out of V Fib/Pulseless VT. Maximal energy (i.e., **360 joules**) should be used for this 4th countershock attempt:

    - Wait about 30-60 seconds (at least) following administration of medication (such as Epinephrine or Lidocaine) *before* proceeding with defibrillation. During this time perform CPR with the goal of circulating medication for optimal effect prior to defibrillation.

    - Deliver either a single shock- or give another *stacked* sequence (i.e., a *second* set of three rapidly delivered shocks with 200-360 joules- *without* any pause between shock attempts for a pulse check).

Refractory V Fib: _Medications of Probable Benefit_

V Fib/Pulseless VT that fails to respond to the measures described in Figure 1B-1 is referred to as _"refractory"_. Lack of response to an initial defibrillation series (of 3 successive shocks), intubation and ventilation, administration of Epinephrine, and a 4th (or 4th, 5th, and 6th) shock is indication for a trial of **antifibrillatory therapy** (Figure 1B-2).

- **Lidocaine** is generally accepted as the _initial_ antifibrillatory agent of choice for medical treatment of refractory V Fib. The recommended dose is **1.0-1.5 mg/kg** ($\approx$50-150 mg) as an _initial_ IV bolus- which may then be repeated in 3-5 minutes.

> **Note**- AHA Guidelines now allow for administration of a **single IV dose** of **1.5 mg/kg** (or $\approx$75-150 mg) of **Lidocaine** in cardiac arrest. Because clearance of this drug is markedly decreased in the arrested heart- continuous IV infusion of Lidocaine need _not_ be started for as long as the patient remains in V Fib.
>
> It should be emphasized that _as soon as_ the patient is converted _out of_ V Fib- Lidocaine pharmacokinetics will change. At this time, _prophylactic_ antiarrhythmic infusion (with either Lidocaine and/or Bretylium) will need to be started (_See below_).

- Following administration of Lidocaine- _defibrillation_ should be repeated (using 360 joules). Wait at least 30-60 seconds after giving the drug before shocking (during which time CPR is performed).

- If V Fib persists after giving Lidocaine- consider **Bretylium**. Practically speaking, if a single IV bolus of Lidocaine is not effective- in most cases a second IV bolus will _not_ fare much better. Thus, although AHA Guidelines allow for additional Lidocaine- _other_ therapeutic measures (i.e., Bretylium, Magnesium) should be strongly considered at this time.

> **Note**- Another reason to move on to Bretylium
> if a single IV bolus of Lidocaine fails to convert V Fib
> is that *combined* use of these drugs may produce a
> *synergistic* antifibrillatory effect (AHA Text- Pg 7-7).

■ The recommended *initial* IV dose of **Bretylium** for treatment of refractory V Fib is a bolus of 5 mg/kg.
Considering the empiric nature of dosing this drug in
the setting of cardiac arrest (and in the interest of
facilitating calculations in this situation)- we favor
administration of one complete ampule (= **500 mg**)
for the **initial IV bolus** (rather than strict calculation
on a bodyweight basis).

- Circulate the drug (by performing CPR) for 30-60
seconds after giving Bretylium. Then *defibrillate* the patient again.

- If the initial bolus of Bretylium fails to convert the
rhythm- a **2nd IV bolus** of Bretylium (now
using 10 mg/kg- or ≈**1-2 ampules**) may be
tried several minutes later. Additional (10
mg/kg) boluses of Bretylium may be given as
needed (up to a *total* dose of 30-35 mg/kg).

> **Note**- The onset of action of **Bretylium** may be
> *delayed* (for several minutes if treating V Fib- and for
> *as long as* 10-20 minutes if treating VT!). It is there-
> fore important *not* to abandon resuscitative efforts
> until the drug has adequate opportunity to work.

Figure 1B-2- *Treatment Algorithm for*
Refractory V Fib (Cont'd from Figure 1B-1)

Persistence of V Fib/Pulseless VT

■ The patient has *not* responded to:

> - *Shock* (X3)- *Intubation* (and ventilation)-
> - *Epinephrine*- and *shock* again

> This defines the condition as **refractory V Fib**. A trial
> of **antifibrillatory** therapy is now in order.

❖ *Consider **Medications** of **Probable Benefit**:*

■ **Lidocaine:** *(p. 26)*
  - Give **1.0-1.5 mg/kg** (≈50-150 mg) as an initial bolus by IV
    push. May repeat in 3-5 minutes- *although a single dose*
    (at 1.5 mg/kg) *IS acceptable in cardiac arrest.*
  - Resume CPR for 30-60 seconds after giving Lidocaine- *then
    shock again.*

> AHA Guidelines recommend **Lidocaine** as the *antifib-*
> *rillatory agent of choice* for treatment of refractory V Fib.
> The drug need *not* be given as a continuous IV infusion-
> *until* the patient is converted out of V Fib (at which time a
> **prophylactic IV infusion** should be started).

IF Lidocaine is ineffective- then consider:

■ **Bretylium:** *(p. 27)*
  - Give 5 mg/kg (*or a single* **500 mg** IV bolus ≈1 amp)-
    resume CPR for 30-60 seconds- *and then shock
    again.*
  - A 2nd IV bolus (of 10 mg/kg- *or* ≈1-2 amps) may be given
    in 5 minutes if V Fib persists (up to a total dose of
    30-35 mg/kg).

■ May also use **Magnesium:** *(p. 29)*
  - Give **1-2 gm** by IV push- especially for patients with
    known (or suspected) *hypomagnesemia* and/or
    Torsade de Pointes.

■ Search for a **Cause** of the Arrest (i.e., **D**ifferential
  Diagnosis) *(pp. 30-31)*

■ Consideration of **Other Measures** *(pp. 31-34)*

■ <u>If V Fib persists</u>- consider **Magnesium Sulfate**. When used to treat V Fib- AHA Guidelines recommend giving **1-2 g** of the drug by **IV push** (AHA Text- Pg 1-20). This dose may be repeated in 5-10 minutes if there is no response. More gradual dosing (i.e., giving 1-2 g over several minutes, or longer) is suggested for treatment of cardiac arrhythmias with less immediate hemodynamic consequences.

Note- The role of Magnesium Sulfate in the treatment of cardiac arrest is *not* yet completely clear. As a result, use of the drug in this setting is still largely empiric. Although one might intuitively expect patients with low serum magnesium levels to benefit most from this form of therapy- serum levels do *not* necessarily correlate with body stores of this cation. Moreover, a beneficial antiarrhythmic effect has been shown to occur in some patients *despite* normal serum magnesium levels at the time of administration. We therefore suggest the following approach:

- Give the drug to patients in cardiac arrest who are *known* (or at least strongly suspected) to be hypomagnesemic (AHA Text- Pg 1-20). Consider its use also for hypomagnesemic patients with cardiac arrhythmias who are *not* in cardiac arrest- especially when these arrhythmias have been refractory to other treatment. Keep in mind that if the rhythm is *Torsade de Pointes*- Magnesium is clearly the treatment of choice.

- Remember that serum magnesium levels do *not* tell the whole story. Serum levels merely reflect *extracellular* magnesium. Because the over- whelming majority of body magnesium stores are contained within the *intracellular* compart- ment- the serum level may sometimes be nor- mal despite significant *intracellular* (and *intra- myocardial*) magnesium depletion.

- Certain clinical conditions are commonly associated with *intracellular* magnesium depletion- *regardless* of whether or not the serum mag- nesium level falls within the normal range. These conditions include:

  i) *Other electrolyte abnormalities* (especially hypokalemia, hyponatremia, hypocal- cemia, and hypophosphatemia).
  ii) Acute myocardial infarction and cardiac arrest.
  iii) Patients receiving Digoxin or diuretic ther- apy.
  iv) Patients with a history of alcohol abuse or renal impairment.

- The risk of toxicity from giving Magnesium Sulfate to a patient in cardiac arrest is *minimal* (if not negligible)- regardless of whether the prear- rest serum magnesium level is normal or low. As a result- **empiric administration** of **Magnesium** would seem to be *reasonable* (if not advisable) in certain life-threatening clini- cal situations (such as V Fib or sustained VT)- especially if standard measures have already been tried and failed. Empiric administration of Magnesium is reasonable when the serum level of this cation is unavailable or normal in such situations- and especially advised when the serum magnesium level is low or suspected to be low.

▪ If V Fib persists- consider **other** **factors** that could account for the patient's refractory condition. This might include a problem with the **ABCs** (i.e., a non- patent airway, asymmetric or absent breath sounds, lack of a pulse with CPR)- and/or **some other** **pre- disposing cause**:

- _Potentially correctable_ causes of refractory V Fib-
include underlying metabolic disturbance
(such as diabetic ketoacidosis or hyperkalemia), hypothermia, hypovolemia, drug
overdose (especially of cocaine, tricyclic antidepressants, or narcotics)- and/or development of a complication of CPR (such as tension pneumothorax or pericardial tamponade).

- V Fib may also be the end result (i.e., _caused_ by)
many other kinds of processes- such as cardiogenic shock (from extensive myocardial
infarction), massive pulmonary embolism,
ruptured aortic aneurysm, or severe trauma
with exsanguinating hemorrhage. Practically
speaking- specific diagnosis of these types of
conditions is much _less_ important clinically
because of the _improbability_ that V Fib result-
ing from _any_ of these conditions will be
amenable to _any_ form of treatment at this
point in the code.

- Although a predisposing, potentially correctable
cause of refractory V Fib will _not_ be found in
most cases of cardiac arrest- it is still important to _always_ keep this possibility in mind.
This is because if such a cause does exist-
standard treatment measures are _unlikely_ to
be effective unless (and _until_) the predisposing cause can be identified _and_ corrected.

Refractory V Fib: _Other Measures to Consider_

Clinically, it may be helpful to realize that if V Fib persists
despite implementation of the actions listed in Figures 1B-1 and
1B-2- that remaining therapeutic options are relatively limited.
There simply is not that much more that can be done. At this point
in the process, we suggest consideration of the following measures:

- Continuing **Epinephrine**. Recovery from prolonged cardiopulmonary arrest is unlikely unless coronary perfusion pressure (CPP) is adequate (i.e., ≥ 15 mm Hg).
In the arrested heart- it appears that Epinephrine is

needed in *sufficient amount* to achieve such pres-
sures. As a result, the drug should be repeated *at
least* every 3-5 minutes for as long as the patient
remains in cardiac arrest. Consideration might also
be given to increasing the dose of Epinephrine (i.e., to
HDE) if the patient fails to respond to SDE doses.

■ *Considering* **Sodium Bicarbonate**. Although Sodium
Bicarbonate has been freely used in the past for the
treatment of cardiac arrest, recent data strongly
question this practice. In fact, a strong case could be
made for *never* administering any Sodium
Bicarbonate at all during cardiopulmonary resuscita-
tion- *regardless* of what the pH value happens to be.
Instead, efforts at correcting acidosis are probably
better directed at *optimizing ventilation*- especially
during the early minutes of a code when the major
component of acidosis is likely to be *respiratory* in
nature (from **hypo**ventilation). Practically speaking,
acceptable indications for use of Sodium Bicarbonate
in the setting of cardiac arrest are limited. They
include:

  - Severe *metabolic acidosis* (usually to a pH value
      of *less* than 7.20)- that persists beyond
      the initial phase (i.e., *beyond* the first 5-
      15 minutes) of the arrest.

  - Cardiac arrest in a patient *known* to have a
      severe *preexisting* metabolic acidosis *prior*
      to the arrest-

      - *IF* any Bicarb is indicated at all dur-
      ing cardiac arrest . . . .

Note- A number of *special* resuscitation situations exist in which use of Bicarb is both appropriate and *likely* to be helpful. These include hyperkalemia and drug overdose with tricyclic antidepressants or phenobarbital (AHA Text- Pg 7-15).

■ **Repeat Countershock** *as needed*. Practically speaking,
there is *no limit* to the number of times that a patient
can be defibrillated. As long as V Fib persists- a

potentially treatable situation is present. After every intervention, CPR should be performed (for a period of at least 30-60 seconds) to allow time for drug to reach the central circulation- and this should then be followed by *repeat countershock* (at an energy level of between 200-360 joules)- until there is conclusive evidence of cardiovascular unresponsiveness.

KEY- It is essential to *always* check for a pulse after *every* intervention- and/or *whenever* the rhythm changes on the monitor. Forgetting to do so may result in iatrogenic defibrillation of a patient in sinus rhythm whose monitor leads fell off. (The *only* exception to this rule is between shocks in a given *stacked* defibrillation series.)

■ *IV **Beta-Blockers**.* The most difficult part about suggesting recommendations for the use of IV beta-blockers in the setting of cardiopulmonary arrest is knowing when to administer these drugs. Clearly, most resuscitation attempts will *not* need IV beta-blockers. However, there *may* be times when all other treatment measures will fail- and *only* IV beta-blockers will save the patient.

Situations in which the use of an IV beta-blocker is most likely to be potentially lifesaving are those in which excessive *sympathetic* tone is implicated as an important etiologic factor in the arrest. Such situations include the following:

- A *prearrest* setting of known ischemia and/or acute *anterior* infarction (especially when cardiac arrest is preceded by a period of tachycardia or hypertension).

- Cardiac arrest that occurs in association with *drug overdose* (from either cocaine or amphetamines).

- Severe stress or anxiety during the prearrest period.

We suggest you consider **empiric use** of an **IV beta-blocker** if *refractory* V Fib occurs in association with any of the above factors- especially if other antiarrhythmic agents have failed (and/or sinus tachycardia appears to precede each recurrence). Because of ease of administration and familiarity with its use- ***Propranolol*** is the IV beta-blocker most commonly selected for treatment of patients in cardiac arrest.

- The recommended dose of Propranolol is to give **0.5-1.0 mg** by ***slow*** **IV** administration (i.e., *not to exceed 1 mg/minute!*). This dose may be repeated (if/as needed)- up to a total dose of 3-5 mg.

- Alternatively, *other* IV beta-blockers (i.e., Esmolol, Atenolol, Metoprolol) could be used instead of Propranolol.

■ ***Procainamide***. AHA Guidelines list Procainamide as a medication "of probable benefit for treatment of persistent/recurrent V Fib". However, they also acknowledge that Procainamide is *rarely* used for this purpose *"because of the prolonged time required to administer effective doses"* (AHA Text- Pg 7-8). We share these reservations about the use of Procainamide as an antifibrillatory agent, and question its efficacy in this setting. *Other* measures should probably be considered first.

■ ***Amiodarone***. Amiodarone is a class III antiarrhythmic agent. Although the drug is remarkably effective as an oral agent in the long-term management of supraventricular and ventricular arrhythmias- experience with use of IV Amiodarone in the setting of cardiac arrest is limited. However, initial experience is encouraging, and it appears that IV Amiodarone may provide a more effective alternative than either Lidocaine or Bretylium for antifibrillatory therapy in this setting.

Note- IV Amiodarone has recently been approved by the FDA for general use. Although *not* yet included in AHA Guidelines- the drug holds promise of filling an important role in the treatment of *refractory* V Fib that has *not* responded to other measures, as well as for the patient in cardiac arrest from recurrent VT who is not able to maintain sinus rhythm with conventional therapy. Time will determine the ultimate role of this newly approved drug.

IF (*As Soon As*) the Patient is Converted *Out of* V Fib

It is important to emphasize the need to *immediately* start a **prophylactic IV infusion** of an **antiarrhythmic agent** as soon as the patient is converted out of V Fib/Pulseless VT. Failure to do so may result in recurrence of the cardiac arrest. AHA Guidelines advise beginning IV infusion with *that* antiarrhythmic agent *"that appeared to aid in the restoration of a pulse"* (AHA Text- Pg 1-20).

In most cases, the appropriate antiarrhythmic agent to use will be **Lidocaine**. If bolus therapy has *not* yet been given (and/or if more than 5 minutes have elapsed since the time of the last Lidocaine dose)- then an **IV bolus** (of **50-100 mg**) should also be administered when the IV infusion is started.

- For the patient with a spontaneous rhythm- the usual *range* for an IV infusion of Lidocaine is between 0.5-4 mg/minute. Practically speaking, most patients will be adequately treated at infusion rates of between 1-2 mg/minute.

- Lower infusion rates (of 0.5-1 mg/minute) are advised for patients at greater risk of developing Lidocaine toxicity. Such patients include the elderly and patients with heart failure, liver disease, or shock. In the *absence* of these factors- we suggest **beginning** the **prophylactic IV infusion** of **Lidocaine** at a rate of **2 mg/minute**. To minimize the risk of developing Lidocaine toxicity, we suggest avoidance of higher infusion rates if at all possible.

***Note*-** We have already emphasized how Lidocaine pharmacokinetics are markedly altered in the arrested heart. Clearance of this drug is significantly *decreased* in this situation- so that as little as one (or *at most* two) boluses of Lidocaine will usually be enough to maintain adequate therapeutic levels *without* the need for continuous IV infusion. As a result, AHA Guidelines recommend *withholding* initiation of a maintenance IV infusion until *after* the patient is converted out of V Fib (AHA Text-Pg 1-19).

Our practice differs slightly from that recommended by AHA Guidelines. Instead of delaying IV infusion of Lidocaine until after the patient is converted out of V Fib- we prefer to initiate an IV infusion while the patient is *still in* cardiac arrest. Our reason for doing so is that we feel it far simpler to *always* initiate the maintenance infusion *at the same time* the decision is made to administer IV loading boluses- even during the low-flow state of cardiac arrest. Pharmacokinetically, this practice should *not* pose a significant risk of developing drug toxicity- since the amount of drug administered at an infusion rate of 2 mg/minute during a 15- to 30-minute resuscitation effort will not exceed 30 to 60 mg. On the other hand, stopping (or never starting) the Lidocaine infusion during the period of cardiac arrest makes it all too easy to forget to immediately start (or restart) the infusion after conversion out of V Fib- which would substantially increase the risk of recurrence.

Bottom Line- It should be equally acceptable to *either* begin the IV infusion of Lidocaine *while* the patient is still in V Fib- or to *defer* this action until *after* the patient is converted out of V Fib. The point to emphasize is that if you choose *not* to begin the Lidocaine maintenance infusion at the time you administer one or more loading boluses of the drug- it is *imperative* to remember to do so *as soon as* the patient is converted *out of* V Fib.

Lidocaine is clearly the most commonly used antifibrillatory agent in the setting of cardiac arrest- as well as the drug most commonly selected for prophylactic IV infusion to prevent V Fib recurrence. However, it should be realized that this drug is *not* necessarily the optimal agent for this purpose in all patients. Although it will often be admittedly difficult in the setting of cardiac arrest to determine which drug(s) or actions are directly responsible for a beneficial (or detrimental) clinical response by the patient- there are times when Lidocaine will fail, and the patient will seemingly *only* be converted out of V Fib after use of **Bretylium**. In such cases, the *prophylactic* approach to prevent V Fib recurrence may differ from that stated above. We suggest consideration of the following points:

- Because the duration of action from an **IV bolus** of **Bretylium** is relatively prolonged (usually lasting 2-6 hours)- some protection against immediate recurrence of V Fib is automatically provided by this form of administration.

- Additional protection against V Fib recurrence may be afforded by starting an IV infusion of **Lidocaine** (after appropriate bolus therapy)- *as suggested above.*

- *Alternatively*- selecting a prophylactic **IV infusion** of **Bretylium** (at a rate of between **1-2 mg/minute**) may be preferred to Lidocaine when this antifibrillatory agent is effective in converting V Fib after Lidocaine has failed. Rarely, IV infusion of both agents may be needed. As already noted- AHA Guidelines advise use of *that* antiarrhythmic agent *"that appears to aid in the restoration of a pulse".*

V Fib/Pulseless VT: *Special Situations* in Resuscitation

Special considerations are needed for treatment of cardiac arrest that occurs in association with the following situations (AHA Text- Pg 1-16):

- If a **Nitroglycerin patch** is on the victim's chest. Remove the patch *prior* to defibrillation (or at least make sure the defibrillator paddle does *not* touch the patch). Practically speaking, the nitroglycerin in the patch will not "explode"- although it may *smoke*, produce *visible arcing*, or *burn* the patient if it comes in contact with the electrical discharge.

■ If the victim has either an *implanted **pacemaker** or **ICD**
(**I**mplanted **C**ardioverter-**D**efibrillator)*. Avoid placement of the defibrillator paddles or pads directly over
(or close to) the generator unit of the device. Passage
of current in close proximity to the unit may severely
damage or lead to misprogramming of the pacemaker
or ICD.

■ If the victim is **hypothermic**. Continued defibrillation
(i.e., *after* the initial series of the first 3 shocks) is *not*
indicated when the patient is hypothermic. Instead,
the hypothermic victim who *remains* in V Fib/
Pulseless VT should be **rewarmed** *before* delivery of
additional shocks.

Note- In our experience- body temperature is the
most *neglected* vital sign in the setting of cardiac
arrest. Typically, no mention at all is made in the
resuscitation record of the patient's body temperature
either before or during the arrest. Be aware that
hypothermia occurs more often than is commonly
appreciated- and may be unsuspected. Hypothermia
may occur even in warm weather states during warm
weather months- especially if the patient is predis-
posed to developing hypothermia (because of being
elderly, debilitated, alcoholic, and/or septic).

Questions to Further Understanding

What Energy is Optimal for Defibrillation?

Although the current recommendation for defibrillation of
adults on the initial countershock attempt is 200 joules- this is
not necessarily the optimal energy level for all patients.
Defibrillation is not benign. On the contrary, use of excessive
energy with countershock attempts can sometimes produce an
adverse result (in the form of additional conduction system damage and/or conversion of V Fib to asystole).

When transthoracic resistance (TTR) values are low, as little
as 100 joules will successfully defibrillate the overwhelming
majority of patients. Use of excessive energy in such individuals
(i.e., 300 or more joules) is likely to be *counterproductive* and

result in a decreased chance of converting the patient out of V Fib. In contrast, higher energy levels (of *at least* 300-360 joules) are much more likely to be needed for defibrillation to be successful when TTR is high. The problem is that *there is no practical way to determine TTR at the moment of countershock delivery with the types of defibrillators in current use.* Until **current-based defibrillators** (that are able to *instantaneously* measure TTR, and adjust current delivery accordingly) become generally available, *empiric* use of **200 joules** for the initial countershock attempt in adults may represent the most reasonable compromise.

What Energy to Use if V Fib Recurs Later On in the Code?

If V Fib *recurs* at a later point in the code (i.e., in a patient who has already been defibrillated *out of* V Fib)- AHA Guidelines advise that *"shocks should be reinitiated at the energy level that previously resulted in successful defibrillation"* (AHA Text- Pg 4-6). While fully acknowledging this recommendation, we nevertheless prefer to *drop back* to **200 joules** in most cases because:

i) Defibrillation is *not* benign. Use of excessive energy can clearly produce conduction system damage- and even asystole.

ii) Just because a patient fails to respond to 200 joules at an earlier point in the code does *not* necessarily mean that they won't respond to this same energy at a *later* point in the code (i.e, *after* oxygenation, administration of Epinephrine and antiarrhythmic medication, correction of electrolyte and acid-base abnormalities, etc.).

The approach we suggest to this issue is simple: If the patient fails to respond to repeat defibrillation at the lowered energy level (i.e., of 200 joules)- *increase* the energy level (to 360 joules)- *and defibrillate again.* Little time should be lost by this approach- and it should allow defibrillation to be accomplished at the *lowest* possible energy level.

> **Bottom Line**- Selection of an energy level of *either* **200** *or* **360 joules** is probably appropriate for the initial attempt at *repeat* defibrillation. If the lower energy level is selected but is unsuccessful- the next repeat attempt should be with 360 joules.
>
> Alternatively, one might begin repeat defibrillation at an intermediate energy level (i.e., of 300 joules)- increasing this to 360 joules if V Fib persists.

Should a Precordial Thump be Used?

Although the precordial thump may occasionally convert a patient out of either VT or V Fib- the maneuver appears to be much more likely to either have no effect, or to exacerbate the rhythm (i.e., precipitate a pulseless rhythm or produce asystole). This is because the emergency care provider has absolutely no control over when in the cardiac cycle the energy will be delivered with the thump. Aggravation of the rhythm is likely if the thump is inadvertently delivered during the vulnerable period.

Clinically- we find it easiest to think of the thump as a *"No-Lose" Procedure*. We therefore generally reserve use of the thump for treatment of rhythms *without* a pulse- *since there is really "nothing to lose" from treatment of such rhythms.* In contrast, we are *against* using the thump to treat a patient in sustained VT in which a pulse is present- since there is "too much to lose" in this situation (i.e., you may lose the pulse). Programmed delivery of an electrical impulse at a *designated* point in the cardiac cycle (i.e., use of *synchronized cardioversion*) is a far more preferable form of treatment for sustained VT associated with a palpable pulse.

Other instances in which the use of a precordial thump is reasonable include treatment of *pulseless* VT and/or V Fib. Practically speaking, however, if a defibrillator is readily available (or will *very soon* be available)- we feel it is equally reasonable to withhold the thump in favor of delivery of an electrical impulse (i.e., defibrillation).

Will Prompt Defibrillation Cause Asystole?

Admittedly, shocking a patient in ventricular fibrillation _does_ run the risk of precipitating asystole- _especially_ if the patient has been in V Fib for a period of time. Nevertheless, the overall likelihood that a patient in V Fib will ultimately survive appears to be significantly greater if they are _immediately_ defibrillated (i.e., _before_ attempting intubation and/or drug administration!)- than if these other interventions are attempted first.

> **_KEY_**- It is important to appreciate that the _realistic_ chance for meaningful (i.e., neurologically intact) _long-term survival_ is relatively small when a patient is found in out-of-hospital cardiac arrest with V Fib as the initial mechanism. Nevertheless, a _chance_ for survival _is_ there- and it is _maximized_ by immediately defibrillating the patient _as soon as this is possible_ (i.e., _before_ attempting intubation and/or drug administration).

What to Remember about CPR?

CPR- in and of itself- will unfortunately _not_ prevent V Fib from deteriorating to asystole. However, performance of CPR may _delay_ deterioration of the rhythm to asystole- and in so doing preserve the period of _viability_ (i.e., _potential_ responsiveness to defibrillation) for a short amount of time (of perhaps 1-2 minutes?).

Although the precise mechanism of CPR remains uncertain (and _several_ mechanisms may be operative at the same time to varying degrees)- what _does_ seem clear is that the efficacy of CPR can be enhanced by attention to _four_ factors:

i) _Compressing with proper form and sufficient force_- not "ribbreaking" force, but enough force to adequately depress the sternum.

ii) _Compressing at the higher end of the recommended rate range_- or as close to 100 compressions/minute as possible.

iii) _Giving Epinephrine ASAP during resuscitation_- since this is the _KEY_ drug for favoring blood flow to the coronary and cerebral circulations.

iv) _Optimizing ventilation_- being sure to deliver slow, full respirations.

Which Route is Best for Giving Drugs?

A **central line** inserted *above* the diaphragm (i.e., a *subclavian* or *internal jugular* line) is the optimal route for drug delivery during cardiac arrest (assuming a provider is present who can rapidly insert the line with a minimal chance of causing pneumothorax). In contrast, a *femoral line* is an ineffective route for drug delivery in the arrested heart (unless a long enough catheter is used that can be threaded *above* the diaphragm).

> **Note**- The **ET route** is an excellent alternative option (and the access route of choice) for medication administration in patients who are intubated *before* IV access is acheived. It should be noted that higher than usual doses of Epinephrine (2-3 times the peripheral dose- *or more!*) may be needed when this drug (or any other drug) is administered by the ET route.

In the absence of a central line, use of a **peripheral IV** may be adequate in most cases of cardiac arrest provided:

  i) a *large bore* IV catheter is used
  ii) a *proximal* site (such as the anticubital fossa) is chosen
      for insertion.

Drug delivery from a peripheral IV during cardiopulmonary resuscitation may further be optimized by:

  iii) *flushing the IV line* (with 50-100 ml of fluid)
  iv) *raising the arm* after drug administration.

In contrast to establishment of a large bore peripheral IV-placement of a small "butterfly" in the dorsum of the wrist will *not* be an effective route for drug administration in the arrested heart.

> **Bottom Line**- *Use whatever access route is established first.* If this happens to be a central line *above* the diaphragm- continue to administer drugs (such as Epinephrine) by this route. If instead, it is a peripheral IV line- our preference is to follow with the next dose of Epinephrine by the ET route (as soon as the patient is intubated). On the other hand, if the ET route is established first- we'll tend to follow with the next dose of Epinephrine by peripheral IV (as soon as the line is inserted).

Which Drugs Can Be Given by the ET Route?

The drugs that *can* be given by the ET route are easily remembered with the assistance of one or more mnemonics:

- **A L E** - **A**tropine, **L**idocaine, and **E**pinephrine.

- **A L O E** - **A**tropine, **L**idocaine, **O**xygen (which *is* a drug), and **E**pinephrine.

- **N A V E L** - **N**arcan (for cardiac arrest due to narcotic overdose), **A**tropine, **V**alium (if seizures accompany the arrest), **E**pinephrine, and **L**idocaine.

Is There an Easy Way to Remember How to Prepare IV Infusions?

Use of the **"Rule of 250 ml"** greatly facilitates recall of an easy-to-learn method for estimating the appropriate *initial* IV infusion rate for *most* of the essential drugs used in ACLS. Adjustments in dosing can then be made based on the patient's clinical response. The rule is as follows:

> Mix **1 unit** of *whatever* drug you are using in **250 ml** of D5W- and set the IV infusion to run at **15-30 drops/minute**.

The *KEY* to application of the **"Rule of 250 ml"** lies with determining the amount of drug contained in one "unit". *Our calculations assume the following:*

For the *antiarrhythmic agents,* **1 unit of drug** = 1 g of **Lidocaine**.
= 1 g of **Procainamide**.
= 1 g of **Bretylium**.
For the *catecholamines,*
1 unit of drug = 1 mg (= 1 vial) of **Isoproterenol**.
= 1 mg (=1 ampule) of **Epinephrine** (in a 1:10,000 concentration for **SDE**).

For *Dopamine,* **1 unit of drug** = 200 mg (= 1 ampule) of **Dopamine**.

Substitution into the **Rule of 250 ml** of the quantities listed above for "1 unit" of drug (for any of the three *antiarrhythmic agents,* two *catecholamines,* or for *Dopamine*) automatically results in an appropriately prepared initial IV infusion rate. Thus one might proceed in the following manner to prepare an IV infusion of these drugs:

- **Lidocaine**- Mix **1 g** (= 1 unit) of *Lidocaine* in **250 ml** of D5W (or 2 g in 500 ml), and set the infusion to run at **30 drops/minute** (= 2 mg/minute).

- **Procainamide**- Mix **1 g** (= 1 unit) of *Procainamide* in **250 ml** of D5W (or 2 g in 500 ml), and set the infusion to run at **30 drops/minute** (= 2 mg/minute).

- **Bretylium**- Mix **1 g** (= 1 unit) of *Bretylium* in **250 ml** of D5W (or 2 g in 500 ml), and set the infusion to run at **15 drops/minute** (= 1 mg/minute).

- **Isoproterenol**- Mix **1 mg** (i.e., 1 vial = 1 unit) of *Isoproterenol* in **250 ml** of D5W, and set the infusion to run at **30 drops/minute** (= 2 µg/minute).

- **S**tandard **D**ose **E**pinephrine (**SDE**)- Mix **1 mg** (i.e., 1 ampule = 1 unit) of a *1:10,000 solution of Epinephrine* in **250 ml** of D5W, and set the infusion to run at between **15-30 drops/minute** (= 1-2 µg/minute).

> **Note-** Calculation of an IV infusion of higher dose Epinephrine does *not* follow the *Rule of 250 ml.*

- **Dopamine-** Mix **200 mg** (i.e., 1 ampule = 1 unit) of *Dopamine* in **250 ml** of D5W, and set the infusion to run at between **15-30 drops/minute** ($\approx$ 2-5 μg/kg/minute for most patients).

What is the Maximum Number of Times You Can Defibrillate a Patient?

As already emphasized- *there is no maximum number.* As long as the rhythm is V Fib- the mechanism of cardiac arrest is potentially treatable (and may respond to defibrillation). Search for a *potentially correctable* underlying cause of V Fib, and *continued* administration of Epinephrine, repeat countershock, and additional antifibrillatory measures are indicated- *until* cardiovascular unresponsiveness can be *conclusively* demonstrated.

When Should Resuscitation Efforts be Terminated?

If a patient has remained in V Fib for *more than* 30 minutes *despite* application of appropriate treatment measures (i.e., application of the steps in Figures 1B-1 and 1B-2)- the chance that resuscitation will be successful, *and* that the patient will survive to *ultimately leave the hospital neurologically intact* is exceedingly small (if not negligible!). As a result, we feel it reasonable to declare "cardiovascular unresponsiveness" (and *terminate* resuscitation efforts) *after* this period of time has passed.

> **Note-** Practically speaking, the chance of neurologically intact long-term survival is exceedingly small if the patient fails to respond to appropriate resuscitation efforts after 20 minutes!

Exceptions to this general rule (when you may want to continue resuscitation efforts *beyond* 20-30 minutes) include:

i) Resuscitation of *children* (who may sometimes fully recover after far longer periods of time).
ii) *Hypothermia* (in which a patient should *never* be pronounced dead "until they are *warm* and dead").
iii) Victims of *drowning* (especially *cold water drowning*).
iv) Patients with *recurrent* V Fib (i.e., when the patient goes "in and out" of V Fib *multiple* times).

What Should Be Done After the Code is "Over"?

The checklist of "things to do" at the end of a successful resuscitation effort includes the following:

1) Verify the adequacy of the **A**irway and **B**reathing (i.e., the adequacy of ventilation and oxygenation, the presence of bilateral and symmetric breath sounds, lung excursion, patient color, ABGs, etc.).
2) Verify the adequacy of **C**irculation (i.e., the presence of a pulse, adequacy of blood pressure, intravascular volume status).
3) Consider the **D**ifferential **D**iagnosis- looking for an *identifiable* (and hopefully *correctable*) precipitating *cause* of the arrest.
4) Verify that a **Lidocaine** bolus has been given- and that the patient is on a continuous IV infusion of the drug (and/or of another antifibrillatory agent).
5) Determine what (if any) other medications that the patient is receiving. *Are these other medications still needed?*
6) Be sure "routine" laboratory tests have been ordered including:

- Chest X-ray (for ET tube, central line placement, assessment of hemodynamic status).
- 12-lead ECG (for evidence of acute infarction /ischemia, definitive rhythm determination).
- Blood work (i.e., CBC, SMAC-25, serum electrolytes including serum magnesium, etc.).

7) Be sure the patient's family has been talked to (and that they are satisfied with the explanation of events of the code that was given to them).

8) Is the patient a *candidate* for **thrombolytic therapy**? This question is usually answered by review of the patient's 12-lead ECG- looking for evidence of acute infarction with new ST segment elevation. Keep in mind that thrombolytic therapy *may* still be administered even if the patient has received CPR- provided that the period of chest compression was not prolonged (usually 10 minutes or less).

9) Acknowledge the efforts of your co-workers.

10) Write a note in the chart.

11) Notify the patient's attending physician (if this is not you).

12) Spend a moment reflecting on how things went during the code- *how things might have gone better-* and what you might do differently (if anything) next time.

13) Update the patient's code status (in case they arrest again).

> **Note-** Items #8 through 13 on this list should be done *regardless* of whether or not the resuscitation effort was successful.

Is Long-Term Survival from Out-of-Hospital Cardiac Arrest Likely if EMS/Paramedic Efforts Fail to Restore Spontaneous Circulation On the Scene?

No. Practically speaking, the chances for long-term, neurologically intact survival from out-of-hospital cardiac arrest are exceedingly small if adequately performed BLS and ACLS measures (including defibrillation) fail to restore a spontaneous pulse in the field. This sobering fact provides the rationale for full application of ACLS procedures by trained paramedical personnel *at the scene-* rather than prematurely rushing the pulseless patient to an emergency department.

> **Note**- The opposite situation to cardiac arrest holds true for the victim of severe trauma- for whom expeditious transfer to a capable facility after field stabilization offers the greatest chance for meaningful survival.

The moral is clear. Early defibrillation is the *KEY* determinant of survival from out-of-hospital cardiac arrest. Although every effort *must* always be made to resuscitate a patient (until there is *definitive* evidence of cardiovascular unresponsiveness)- realistic chances for long-term survival are small if properly performed BLS/ACLS in the field fails to restore spontaneous circulation.

Tachycardia

The goal of this section is to present an overall approach to evaluation and management for the patient who is found in **Tachycardia**. Although discussion of *supraventricular* and *ventricular* tachyarrhythmias is usually *not* grouped together- doing so enhances clinical practicality and allows the broadest overview of clinical situations that are likely to be encountered.

The Overview Algorithm for Tachycardia

The approach recommended by AHA Guidelines for the patient with tachycardia is illustrated in <u>Figure 1C-1</u>. Foremost in this approach is determination of whether the patient has a pulse in association with the rhythm.

> ***KEY***- If there is **NO pulse** present in association with the rhythm shown in Figure 1C-1- one would have to interpret this rhythm as **Pulseless VT**. As emphasized in Section 1B, this pulseless condition is treated in the *identical* manner as **V Fib**. Treatment entails **immediate defibrillation** (i.e., *unsynchronized* countershock)- and application of the series of steps and actions described in detail in Figures 1B-1 and 1B-2.

Note that the algorithm shown in Figure 1C-1 assumes that the tachycardia *IS* associated with a pulse. This means that the patient (by definition) is *not* in full cardiac arrest. The *KEY* to management in this situation now lies with determining if the patient in question is hemodynamically stable:

- *If the patient **IS** hemodynamically **STABLE**-* take a deep breath! By definition, there is at least *some* time to proceed with further evaluation. As indicated in Figure 1C-1- subsequent management will depend on *specific* **diagnosis** of the tachyarrhythmia. Four principal entities should be considered. These include:

  i) ***Atrial Fibrillation (A Fib)*** or ***Flutter***
  ii) ***PSVT***
  iii) ***Ventricular Tachycardia (VT)***
  iv) ***W****ide-****C****omplex* ***T****achycardia* (**WCT**) of ***Uncertain* Type**.

  For the patient with tachycardia who is hemodynamically stable- once diagnosis of the *type* of tachycardia is made, a trial of medical therapy can be attempted.

  > **Note**- AHA Guidelines do *not* include **sinus tachycardia** in the overview algorithm for treatment of *Tachycardia* (AHA Text- Pg 1-33). This intentional omission emphasizes the point that the treatment of choice for *sinus tachycardia* is *not* drugs or cardioversion- but rather to *identify* and *correct* the underlying *cause* of the tachycardia.

- *If the patient with tachycardia is **NOT** hemodynamically **STABLE**-* then more immediate treatment is needed. Practically speaking- it *no longer matters* what specific diagnosis of the tachyarrhythmia is, since *immediate* **synchronized cardioversion** will be indicated *regardless* of what the rhythm happens to be.

Figure 1C-1- *Overview Algorithm for Tachycardia*

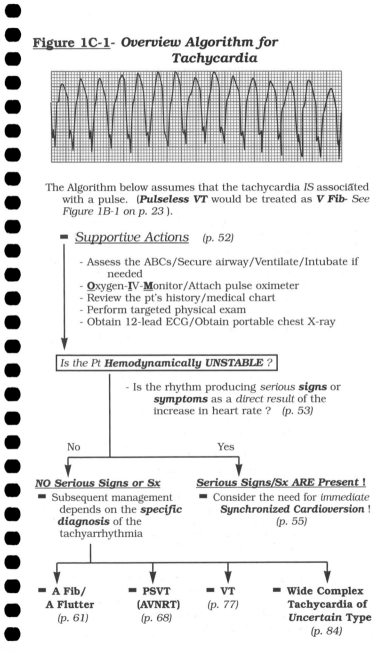

The Algorithm below assumes that the tachycardia *IS* associated with a pulse. (***Pulseless VT*** would be treated as **V Fib**- *See Figure 1B-1 on p. 23*).

■ *Supportive Actions*   (p. 52)

   - Assess the ABCs/Secure airway/Ventilate/Intubate if needed
   - **O**xygen-**I**V-**M**onitor/Attach pulse oximeter
   - Review the pt's history/medical chart
   - Perform targeted physical exam
   - Obtain 12-lead ECG/Obtain portable chest X-ray

*Is the Pt **Hemodynamically UNSTABLE** ?*

   - Is the rhythm producing *serious* **signs** or **symptoms** as a *direct result* of the increase in heart rate ?   (p. 53)

No   Yes

NO *Serious Signs or Sx*   ***Serious Signs/Sx ARE Present* !**
■ Subsequent management   ■ Consider the need for *immediate*
   depends on the **specific**   **Synchronized Cardioversion** !
   diagnosis of the   (p. 55)
   tachyarrhythmia

■ A Fib/   ■ PSVT   ■ VT   ■ Wide Complex
A Flutter   (AVNRT)   (p. 77)   Tachycardia of
(p. 61)   (p. 68)   Uncertain Type
                                                           (p. 84)

> **Note**- AHA Guidelines allow that even when the decision to cardiovert *"immediately"* has been made, medical therapy *may* still be tried- *IF* drugs are *immediately* available- and *provided that* giving these drugs does *not* result in delay of cardioversion (AHA Text- Pg 1-35). Clearly- *clinical judgement is needed at the bedside* in the decision making process.

On the *Sequence* of Actions

Although *not* specifically shown in Figure 1C-1, evaluation of the patient routinely begins with the **Universal Algorithm** (Figure 1A-1 on page-6)- in which *responsiveness* of the victim is first assessed and the **ABC**s are attended to. Other **Supportive Actions** listed are implemented at the earliest appropriate opportunity (depending on resources and the number and skills of available rescuers).

- The **Supportive Actions** listed in Figure 1C-1 are similar to those that should be implemented in virtually *all* of the ACLS algorithms for treatment. As noted above- these actions are implemented at the *earliest appropriate* opportunity.

- AHA Guidelines fully acknowledge that "astute clinicians" *cannot* progress slowly (i.e., *step-by-step*) through every intervention in each recommended sequence for the brady- and tachyarrhythmias (AHA Text- Pg 1-30). Thus *despite* being listed separately- many interventions are really performed *simultaneously* in practice, and sometimes in a sequence that is *modified* from that given in the algorithms. For example, synchronized cardioversion may *need* to be performed *before* some of the *Supportive Actions* that are listed in Figure 1C-1- *especially* if the patient is hemodynamically unstable.

> **Note**- If the patient decompensates at *any* time- *STOP* treatment. *Immediately* **cardiovert** the patient. Administration of drugs is of *secondary* importance if the patient is (or at *any* time becomes) hemodynamically unstable.

Is Synchronized Cardioversion *Acutely* Needed?

The purpose of *synchronization* is to deliver the electrical impulse at a point in the cardiac cycle (i.e., at the peak of the QRS complex) when the heart is *least "vulnerable"* to precipitation of V Fib. Cardioversion of *organized* tachyarrhythmias is generally *much safer* when synchronization is used.

The principal indication for use of *synchronized* cardioversion is in the treatment of **tachyarrhythmias** (including *both* VT and *SUPRAventricular* rhythms) that are either hemodynamically *unstable*- and/or which fail to respond to other measures. Clinically, cardioversion is needed *emergently* only if the patient *is* (and/or *becomes*) acutely unstable. If the patient with tachycardia is *not* acutely unstable- then an initial trial of antiarrhythmic therapy is often preferred. Cardioversion may still be needed *later* in some of these patients (i.e., if medical therapy fails to control the rhythm)- but in such cases it can usually be performed under less urgent conditions (i.e., there should at least be time to *sedate* the patient and call anesthesia to the bedside).

> **Note**- The decision of whether or not to *immediately* cardiovert a patient may sometimes have to be made *before* determining the specific diagnosis of the tachyarrhythmia! As we have already emphasized, if the patient is *hemodynamically unstable*- knowing the specific arrhythmia diagnosis *no longer matters*. The *critical* therapeutic question to ask first then, in assessing the patient with tachycardia- is *whether or not* to perform synchronized cardioversion (AHA Text- Pg 1-32).

- *Is the rhythm **hemodynamically significant?*** A brady- or tachyarrhythmia *becomes* hemodynamically significant- *IF* the rhythm produces *serious **signs** or **symptoms*** as a *direct result* of the reduction (or increase) in heart rate. For the purpose of this definition:

    - ***Signs of Concern***- include hypotension (i.e., systolic BP ≤80-90 mm Hg), shock, heart failure/pulmonary edema, and/or Acute MI.

    - ***Symptoms of Concern***- include chest pain, shortness of breath, and/ or decreased mental status.

> **Note**- It is important to emphasize that the definition of *hemodynamic stability* is equally applicable for *SUPRAventricular* tachyarrhythmias- as it is for VT. Thus, a patient with tachycardia who is hypotensive, having chest pain, and mentally confused is probably in need of immediate cardioversion- *regardless* of what the rhythm happens to be. On the other hand, if the patient with tachycardia is *asymptomatic* (i.e., normotensive and *without* chest pain, shortness of breath, or mental confusion)- then there probably is time for more careful evaluation and a trial of medical treatment.

- Synchronized cardioversion is *not* indicated when the tachycardia is simply a reflection of the underlying condition. For example, sinus tachycardia that develops in response to severe hypotension, acute infarction, or pulmonary edema should *not* be cardioverted. As already noted, the treatment of choice for sinus tachycardia is to identify and treat the underlying cause.

- AHA Guidelines emphasize that it is highly *unlikely* for synchronized cardioversion to be needed on an *emergent* basis- *IF* the heart rate of the tachycardia is *less* than **150 beats/minute** (AHA Text- Pg 1-33). Tachycardias at relatively "slower" rates (i.e., of *less* than 150 beats/minute) are much *less likely* to produce serious signs or symptoms- especially in patients who have normal ventricular function. Cardioversion might still be needed in some of these patients at a *later* time (i.e., *non-emergently* under more stable conditions)- *IF* medical therapy fails to control/convert the tachyarrhythmia.

■ *Not all patients with sustained VT are (or immediately become) hemodynamically unstable* ! In fact, some patients with VT are able to remain alert and maintain an adequate blood pressure for minutes, hours (*and even days!*)- *without* showing any signs of decompensation. Thus the first thing to do when confronted with a patient who presents in a worrisome looking tachycardia is to:

> i) *Take a DEEP breath!*
> ii) Remember to assess the patient in the manner suggested in Figure 1C-1.

■ Finally- although certain parameters are frequently cited for defining hemodynamic stability (such as a systolic BP of ≥80-90 mm Hg)- *bedside* clinical evaluation is often the *best* way to determine the true need for specific treatment. Simply stated- sometimes *"you just have to be there"*- to make an adequate assessment. For example, a patient in VT may *not* necessarily require immediate cardioversion *despite* an extremely low blood pressure reading (i.e., of 70 systolic)- _IF_ they are *otherwise* alert, comfortable, and asymptomatic.

If Synchronized Cardioversion _IS_ _Immediately_ Needed

AHA Guidelines recommend use of the following **Standard Sequence** of **Energy Levels** for *synchronized* cardioversion of the various tachyarrhythmias (AHA Text- Pg 1-35):

■ _1st Attempt_- **100 joules**

> ■ _IF unsuccessful_- increase energy to **200 joules**- - then to **300**- and finally to **360 joules**.

Several **exceptions** exist to the above general recommendations (i.e., when a different energy selection might be preferable for cardioversion of certain arrhythmias). These exceptions include:

- **Polymorphic VT** (i.e., VT with an *irregular* morphology and rate)- which often requires a *higher* energy level for successful cardioversion. AHA Guidelines suggest *starting* with **200 joules**- which may then need to be increased if the rhythm persists.

- **Atrial Flutter**- which often responds to *lower* energy levels (probably because it is a very *organized* arrhythmia with rapid but very regular atrial activity). AHA Guidelines therefore allow for selection of **50 joules** as the *initial* energy level for attempts at converting A Flutter.

- **Atrial Fibrillation**- which in our experience is also often a relatively difficult rhythm to successfully cardiovert when lower energy levels are used. *We* therefore prefer to *start* with **200 joules** for our *initial* attempt at cardioverting A Fib- and to increase this to 360 joules if a second attempt is needed. Other associated clinical factors (i.e., left atrial size, duration of time that the patient has been in A Fib, persistence or correction of the precipitating cause, etc.)- often determine whether or not the patient with A Fib will respond to cardioversion.

KEY- When attempting to cardiovert a patient- *be sure* that the *SYNCH Mode* is properly engaged- that the machine is *sensing* QRS complexes of the tachycardia (usually indicated by a marker on each R wave that is sensed)- and that both discharge buttons are *simultaneously* depressed by the person who is cardioverting (and *maintained depressed*) until the electrical discharge occurs.

The Patient with Tachycardia:
Differential Diagnosis

The importance of determining the **specific diagnosis** of the tachyarrhythmia is evident from inspection of Figure 1C-1. As shown in this algorithm, once established that the patient with **Tachycardia** is hemodynamically stable- diagnosis of the _type_ of tachycardia becomes the major determinant of what treatment course to follow. Practically speaking, there are _six_ principal entities to consider:

1. Sinus Tachycardia- which (as already noted) is _not_ separately listed on Figure 1C-1.
2. Atrial Fibrillation
3. Atrial Flutter- which is _combined_ with A Fib on Figure 1C-1 (because of its similar therapeutic approach).
4. PSVT
5. Ventricular Tachycardia (VT)
6. _Wide-Complex_ Tachycardia (WCT) of _Uncertain_ Etiology

- Differentiation between these six clinical entities can usually be made with surprising accuracy by attention to the following _five_ factors:

  i) The **rate** of the tachycardia.
  ii) The pattern of **regularity** of the rhythm.
  iii) The **width** of the QRS complex.
  iv) The presence (and nature) of **atrial activity**- and its relation (if any) to the QRS complex.
  v) The **clinical setting** in which the arrhythmia occurs (which will usually be defined by information obtained from the **Supportive Actions** that are listed in Figure 1C-1).

- A _KEY_ clinical distinction to make is determination of whether the tachycardia is **ventricular** or **SUPRAventricular** in etiology. Assessment of the **width** of the **QRS complex** provides the most helpful clue in this determination:

> _Regarding **QRS Duration**_- The QRS complex may normally measure _up to_ **0.10 second** in adults. Since one _large_ box on ECG grid paper corresponds to a duration of 0.20 second- this means that a QRS complex may normally be _up to_ half a large box in duration. Practically speaking then- the QRS complex is said to be **_wide_** if it measures **_more_** than **_half_** a **large box** in duration.

■ If the QRS Complex is **_Narrow_**- then the tachycardia _must_ be **SUPRAventricular** (i.e., originating _at_ or _above_ the AV node). The first _four_ entities that were cited above should then be considered:

1. Sinus Tachycardia
2. Atrial Fibrillation
3. Atrial Flutter
4. PSVT

The most common causes of **_S_**upra**_V_**entricular **_T_**achycardia (**SVT**)

Specific points to keep in mind regarding distinction between these four entities are the following:

- **_Sinus Tachycardia_**- usually easy to recognize by the presence of a normal (i.e., _upright_ in lead II) P wave- that precedes each QRS complex and is "married" to it (i.e., related to each QRS by a fixed PR interval). It is unusual for sinus tachycardia to exceed 150-160 beats/minute in an adult patient who is lying in bed.

- **_A Fib_**- characterized by the _irregular irregularity_ of its ventricular response and the _absence_ of P waves. The irregularity of A Fib usually makes it easy to distinguish this rhythm from the other entities on the list.

- **_A Flutter_**- is recognized by the presence of regular _sawtooth_ atrial activity that most often occurs at an atrial rate of close to 300/minute (250-350/minute range). The most common ventricular response to _untreated_ A Flutter is with 2:1 AV conduction- a fact that typically results in a ventricular response of close to 150/minute (i.e., 300 ÷ 2).

- **PSVT**- is a regular supraventricular tachycardia which lacks normal atrial activity. Subtle retrograde (i.e., negative in lead II) P waves are sometimes seen deforming the terminal portion of the QRS complex.

Note- Attention to the ventricular rate may provide an important clue to the type of SVT. For example, consider a *regular* SVT at a rate of 200 beats/minute. In an adult, this rate would be far too fast for the rhythm to be sinus tachycardia. The rate is *not* consistent with what would be expected for A Flutter in an untreated patient- for whom the ventricular response most often will be close to 150 beats/minute (usual range 140-160/minute). Regularity of the rhythm rules out A Fib. By the process of elimination- a regular SVT at a rate of 200 beats/ minute in an adult will almost certainly be PSVT.

On the other hand- distinction between sinus tachycardia, A Flutter, and PSVT may be much more difficult to make when the ventricular rate of a regular SVT is close to 150 beats/minute (since this rate is consistent with *all* three entities).

■ If the QRS Complex is **Wide**- then it is much more likely that the rhythm is of **ventricular** etiology (i.e., ventricular tachycardia). Compared to the various SVTs- VT is far more likely to be a potentially *life-threatening* arrhythmia.

Note- Although the presence of QRS widening should always suggest VT as the *probable* diagnosis- this finding by itself does *not* rule out the possibility of a supraventricular etiology. This is the reason for adding the category *WCT* of *Uncertain Etiology.*

■ Four important **caveats** should be kept in mind regarding the ECG interpretation of a patient with **tachycardia** and **QRS widening**. They are:

  i) That a portion of the QRS complex may sometimes lie *on the baseline* in a particular monitoring lead. In such cases, the QRS complex may appear to be narrow- *when in fact it is not.* Viewing the tachycardia from *more* than one perspective (i.e., use of additional monitoring leads- and ideally obtaining a 12-lead ECG *during* the tachycardia) should facilitate determining what the *true* width of the QRS complex happens to be.

  ii) That a rhythm *may* be *SUPRAventricular* in etiology *despite* QRS widening- if *either* **aberrant conduction** or **preexisting bundle branch block** is present. Availability of a prior ECG on the patient may provide an invaluable clue to this possibility (i.e., by revealing *preexisting* widening of the QRS complex while the patient was in sinus rhythm).

  iii) That the patient's hemodynamic status is *not at all helpful* in the diagnostic process. For example, some patients in VT may be normotensive and asymptomatic (and *remain* so) for surprisingly *long* periods of time!

  iv) That *regardless* of the patient's hemodynamic status- VT is (*by far!*) the most common cause of a regular wide-complex tachycardia.

Bottom Line- If the QRS complex is wide- *always* **assume VT** until *proven* otherwise. *Treat the patient accordingly.*

Figure 1C-2- *Treatment Algorithm for A Fib/Flutter*
(When the patient is hemodynamically stable)

Lead II

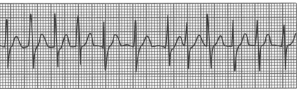

- *Supportive Actions* *(p. 52)*
  - as listed on Figure 1C-1 have *all* been accomplished.

Treatment Options:

- Consider possible *Precipitating CAUSES* of the rhythm: *(p. 62)*
  - *Rule out*- heart failure, Acute MI, hyperthyroidism, hypoxia, pulmonary embolism, alcohol or drug abuse, etc.

- Begin with a *Rate-Slowing* Drug (if the rate is rapid):
  - **Diltiazem** (p. 63)- 0.25 mg/kg (or ≈15-20 mg) initial IV bolus; Follow with 0.35 mg/kg (≈25 mg) in 15 min if no response. May then follow with IV infusion @ 10 mg/hr (5-15 mg/hr range).

    - or -

  - **Verapamil** (p. 64)- 2.5-5 mg IV initially; then 5-10 mg IV.

    - and/or -

  - **Digoxin** (p. 65)- no longer the first drug of choice. Load with 0.25-0.5 mg IV. Then give 0.125-0.25 mg IV q 2-6 hrs (as needed up to 0.75-1.5 mg total).

  - Could also use a **Beta-blocker** (i.e., **IV Propranolol, Esmolol**)- but NOT in close association with IV Verapamil/Diltiazem !!! *(p. 66)*

- Correct *Electrolyte Disturbance* (if present):
  - *Rule out*- hypokalemia, hypomagnesemia.

- Consider Measures to *Convert* the Rhythm: *(p. 67)*
  - Spontaneous conversion to sinus rhythm will often occur if a precipitating cause (*See above*) can be found and corrected.
  - *Medical therapy* (usually **Quinidine** or **Procainamide**).
  - **Synchronized Cardioversion** (performed *non-emergently*).

- Consider the Need for Anticoagulation: *(p. 62)*
  - Use of Heparin/Aspirin (as appropriate).

> **Note**- If the patient decompensates at *any* time during the process of evaluating/treating the tachycardia- *STOP and immediately cardiovert* !

Treatment Algorithm for A Fib/Flutter

The approach we suggest to evaluation and management of the patient in **Atrial Fibrillation** or **Atrial Flutter** is shown in <u>Figure 1C-2</u>.

KEY- For practical purposes- *initial* management of *A Fib* and *A Flutter* in the emergency situation is very similar. That is, the drugs used to achieve rate control and/or convert the rhythm are the same- and synchronized cardioversion is the treatment of choice if the patient becomes acutely unstable. Special points to keep in mind include the following:

i) That it is usually much easier to control the rate of the ventricular response to rapid *A Fib* (i.e., with Digoxin, Verapamil/Diltiazem, or a beta-blocker)- than it is to control the rate of A Flutter.

ii) That *A Flutter* tends to be much more responsive to cardioversion than A Fib (which is why a *lower* initial energy of ≈**50 joules** is usually selected to cardiovert this rhythm)- compared to the **200 joules** that we usually select when attempting to cardiovert *A Fib*.

iii) That the risk of stroke is much higher for A Fib than it is for A Flutter- although anticoagulation will usually *not* be needed in the emergency situation.

Look for an *Underlying* Cause

In addition to rate control of the ventricular response- the *KEY* to successful management of A Fib/Flutter is identification and correction of the *precipitating* condition that caused the rhythm.

■ Common causative conditions include heart failure, Acute MI, hypothyroidism, hypoxia, pulmonary embolism, alcohol or drug abuse (i.e., cocaine), and others.

- Treatment of A Fib/Flutter is much less likely to be successful- *IF* the underlying condition has not been corrected.

> **Note**- In the acute care setting- *neither* A Fib *nor* A Flutter need be treated if the ventricular response is not very rapid (i.e., *less* than ≈110 beats/minute- or so)- and the patient is hemodynamically stable.

When there is a *Rapid* Ventricular Response

Most of the time in the emergency situation- the ventricular response to A Fib/Flutter will be rapid. In this situation, treatment is clearly indicated. Pharmacologic therapy with **rate-slowing drugs** is usually tried first- unless the patient acutely decompensates, in which case synchronized cardioversion should be *immediately* performed.

- **Diltiazem**. IV Diltiazem has clearly become a drug of choice for acute rate control of rapid A Fib/Flutter. Onset of action following IV administration of this agent is fast (i.e., usually *within* 3 minutes of giving an IV bolus)- with peak effect most often occurring by 7 minutes. Effects of an IV bolus generally last 1-3 hours.

  Availability for use as a continuous IV infusion allows for ongoing antiarrhythmic effect over the ensuing 24 hours, and offers a decided advantage compared to other antiarrhythmic agents (such as Digoxin or Verapamil). This is particularly true for *maintaining* rate control over a period of hours when the ventricular response is not readily controlled by intermittent bolus therapy.

  - The recommended dose for the *initial* **IV bolus** of Diltiazem is 0.25 mg/kg (which for an *average-sized* adult is ≈**15-20 mg**). This IV bolus should be given over a 2 minute period.

  - If the desired clinical response is not seen within 15 minutes- a **2nd IV bolus** of approximately **25 mg** (i.e., 0.35 mg/kg) may be given.

- If continued antiarrhythmic effect is desired- a continuous **IV infusion** may be started after bolus administration. The recommended *initial* infusion rate for IV Diltiazem is **10 mg/hr**- which may then be increased to 15 mg/hr (as needed) for clinical effect. IV infusion should generally *not* be continued for more than 24 hours.

> **Note**- It should be emphasized that the above cited doses are for an *average-sized* adult! Significantly *smaller* doses (i.e., of ≈10-15 mg) and *lower* infusion rates (i.e., of 5 mg/hr) should be used for patients of lighter body weight- especially if they are older and/or more likely to have underlying conduction system disease.

- **Verapamil**. Like Diltiazem- Verapamil is a favored drug for emergency treatment of rapid A Fib/Flutter. Although neither of these drugs are very effective for converting A Fib/Flutter to sinus rhythm- both drugs exert a potent AV nodal blocking effect that reliably *slows* the ventricular response.

  - The recommended dose for the *initial* **IV bolus** of Verapamil is **2.5-5 mg** (to be given over a 1-2 minute period). The *lower* amount should be used first, and the drug given more *slowly* (i.e., over 3-4 minutes) to elderly patients and to those with borderline blood pressure. Cautious dosing in this manner should help to minimize the incidence of hypotension and excessive heart rate slowing that may otherwise be seen.

  - Peak effects from an IV bolus of Verapamil are usually seen within 5 minutes.

  - The dose of IV Verapamil may be **repeated** one or more times **after 15-30 minutes** (if/as needed)- up to a *total* dose of ≈30 mg. If the initial dose of 2.5-5 mg is tolerated- then a larger dose (of 5-10 mg) may be given for subsequent IV boluses.

- **Digoxin.** In the acute care setting- both Verapamil and Diltiazem are more effective than Digoxin for *initial* rate control of the ventricular response to A Fib/Flutter. This is because the principal mechanism of action of Digoxin for slowing the rate to A Fib/Flutter is by increasing the amount of vagal tone- which may render the drug less effective in emergency situations in which *sympathetic* tone is tremendously increased.

Bottom Line- Digoxin may work and *can* be used to treat rapid A Fib/Flutter- but IV Diltiazem (or Verapamil) is now preferred and will usually be more effecitve.

Pearl- Combined use of Digoxin and IV Diltiazem/Verapamil may produce a **synergistic effect** in controlling the ventricular response to rapid A Fib/Flutter. Consideration might therefore be given to *adding* Digoxin- if Diltiazem/Verapamil fail to control the ventricular response.

If the decision is made to use Digoxin in the treatment of A Fib/ Flutter- we suggest the following dosing considerations:

- When treating a patient who has not previously received Digoxin- one usually begins with an *initial* **IV loading dose** of **0.25-0.5 mg**. This may be followed with additional **incremental doses** (of **0.125-0.25 mg IV**) that can be given every 2-6 hours as needed (i.e., depending on the ventricular response)- until a *total* loading dose of ≈0.75-1.5 mg of drug has been given. Lower doses may be needed if the drug is used in combination with Diltiazem/Verapamil.

- In the *absence* of hyperthyroidism, hypoxemia, Acute MI, and electrolyte disturbance- the ventricular rate response has been used as an indicator of the adequacy of digitalization. Persistence of a rapid rate after administration of several boluses of Digoxin suggests that additional drug may still be needed to achieve adequate control of the ventricular response. In the presence of any of the above conditions, however, increased sensitivity to the effects of Digoxin (and a correspondingly increased risk of developing toxicity) augurs for much greater caution (and use of lower doses) in administering the drug.

- After IV loading is complete, the patient may be placed on a regular daily maintenance dose (that is usually between 0.125-0.25 mg/day)- if this is appropriate for the clinical situation.

- ◼ **IV Beta-Blockers**. Use of an IV beta-blocker (i.e., **Propranolol**, **Esmolol**- or other) is a perfectly acceptable alternative to IV Diltiazem/Verapamil for emergency treatment of rapid A Fib/Flutter- provided there is no overt heart failure or severe bronchospasm that would contraindicate its use. Practically speaking, IV beta-blockers are not used very often in this setting. This most likely is a reflection of the preference for using IV Diltiazem/Verapamil (and/or Digoxin)- and the fact that IV beta-blockers can *not* be given in close proximity (i.e., with 20-30 minutes) of IV Diltiazem/Verapamil (because combining these agents in this manner could lead to profound bradycardia- and even asystole!).

- ◼ **Synchronized Cardioversion**. Pharmacologic therapy (i.e., with IV Diltiazem/Verapamil and/or Digoxin) is usually preferred for *initial* treatment of rapid A Fib/Flutter when the patient is not acutely unstable. If medical therapy is not effective (and/or the patient becomes hemodynamically unstable *at any time* during the treatment process)- synchronized cardioversion may then be in order:

    - Use **50 joules** for the *initial* attempt at cardioverting **A Flutter**. This will usually be all that is needed.

- Use *more* energy to cardiovert **A Fib**. We suggest selection of **200 joules** for the initial attempt- and then increasing this to 360 joules if the rhythm fails to respond. Realize that A Fib will *not* always respond to synchronized car- dioversion (especially if the underlying cause of the rhythm has not been corrected).

- Synchronized cardioversion is best avoided (if at all possible!) when excessive doses of Digoxin have been administered. Practically speaking, the procedure *can* usually be performed *safely* if the patient has received *therapeutic* doses of Digoxin (and toxicity is *not* present).

Note- IV Diltiazem/Verapamil, Digoxin, and/or beta-blockers are *all* effective drugs for achieving rate control of the ventricular response to rapid A Fib/Flutter. As a result, these drugs (either alone or in combination as described above) constitute the medical treatment of choice for *emergency manage- ment* of these tachyarrhythmias.

Unfortunately- *none* of these agents are more than *minimally* effective for medically converting A Fib/Flutter to normal sinus rhythm. Use of *other* drugs (i.e., Quinidine, Procainamide, Disopyramide, Flecainide, Propafenone, Amiodarone, and/or Sotalol)- and/or *synchronized* cardioversion are clearly far more effective therapeutic interventions for this purpose.

Figure 1C-3- *Treatment Algorithm for PSVT*

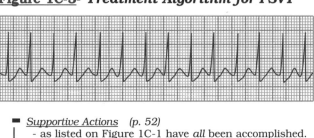

▪ <u>*Supportive Actions*</u>   *(p. 52)*
  - as listed on Figure 1C-1 have *all* been accomplished.

> **_KEY_ Clinical Questions**   *(p. 70)*
>   i) Is the patient hemodynamically stable?
>   ii) Is the QRS complex *truly* narrow?
>   iii) Is the diagnosis *truly* PSVT?

Treatment Options:

▪ <u>Consider the use of a **Vagal Maneuver** :</u>   *(p. 71)*

▪ **<u>Adenosine:</u>**   *(p. 72)*
  - The drug of 1st choice for PSVT (and the drug of
    choice for treatment of *SUPRAventricular* tachy-
    cardias of uncertain etiology).
  - Begin with **6 mg** by *rapid* **IV push** (i.e., over 1-3 sec-
    onds!)- followed by a fluid flush.
  - If no response in 1-2 min, a 2nd dose (of **12 mg**)
    may be given- and repeated if needed in 1-2 min
    (for a total dose of 6 + 12 + 12 = 30 mg).

▪ **<u>Verapamil:</u>**   *(p. 73)*
  - Should only be used if the QRS complex is narrow
    (or the tachycardia is known with *certainty* to be
    PSVT).
  - Give **2.5- 5 mg IV** over 1-2 min; may follow 15-30
    min later with a 2nd dose of 5-10 mg IV. Give
    the drug slower (over 3-4 min) to the elderly.

▪ <u>*Other drugs*</u> that could also be used:
  - **Diltiazem**- comparable effect as Verapamil   *(p. 76)*
  - **Digoxin**- more delayed onset of action   *(p. 75)*
  - **Beta-Blocker**- should *not* be used soon after IV
    Diltiazem/Verapamil !   *(p. 75)*

> **Note**- If the patient decompensates at *any* time
> during the process of evaluating/treating the tachy-
> cardia- *STOP and immediately cardiovert* !

Treatment Algorithm for PSVT

The approach we suggest to evaluation and management of the patient in PSVT is shown in <u>Figure 1C-3</u>. The *KEY* point to emphasize in this approach is the importance of **reentry** as the responsible mechanism in almost all cases. As a result of this phenomenon- a *reentry circuit* is set up, whereby the supraventricular impulse gets caught up in a perpetual cycle in which *after* being conducted to the ventricles, the impulse *returns* to the AV node (in *retrograde* fashion)- before it is once again conducted back down to the ventricles. This process continues until it is either interrupted by treatment or spontaneously resolves.

The goal of therapy for PSVT is to *interrupt* conduction over the reentry circuit. Because each part of the cycle is dependent on the integrity of the previous part- even *momentary* delay in conduction over *any* portion of the circuit may be all that is needed to terminate the arrhythmia. This is the reason special maneuvers such as carotid massage (which only act briefly) may be effective in treatment.

PSVT is known as an **AV nodal dependent** arrhythmia. This is because at least a portion of the reentry circuit almost always involves the AV node. Drugs that affect conduction *through* the AV node (i.e., AV nodal blocking agents such as Diltiazem/Verapamil, Digoxin, and beta-blockers) are therefore effective in treatment.

In contrast to PSVT- A Fib and A Flutter are *not* AV nodal dependent arrhythmias. This means that even though the same AV nodal blocking agents are used in treatment (Figure 1C-2)- these drugs will usually *not* be effective in converting A Fib/Flutter to sinus rhythm. Instead, the primary function of AV nodal blocking drugs in the treatment of A Fib/Flutter is to *slow* the ventricular response of these arrhythmias.

> **Note**- Although we refer to the rhythm shown in Figure 1C-3 as PSVT- many clinicians now prefer the newer term- **AVNRT** (**A**V **N**odal **R**eentry **T**achycardia)- to designate this arrhythmia. The advantage of this newer term is that it more accurately reflects the *mechanism* of this rhythm- which almost always involves **reentry** within (or into) the AV node. For the purpose of consistency with AHA Guidelines, we refer to this rhythm as **PSVT** throughout this Rapid Reference.

Initial Approach: *KEY Clinical Questions*

Before discussing the specific interventions described in Figure 1C-3 for the management of PSVT- three *KEY* clinical questions should be addressed. The importance of considering these questions is best illustrated by applying them to the tachycardia that apppears at the top of Figure 1C-3.

■ Question #1- *Is the patient hemodynamically stable?*

The clinical approach to management of a patient with the rhythm shown clearly depends *first* on hemodynamic status. Only if the patient is hemodynamically stable should further evaluation take place. If the patient is *not* hemodynamically stable- then *immediate* intervention (with synchronized cardioversion *rather than* drugs) should be strongly considered (*See Figure 1C-1*).

If the patient is hemodynamically stable- then there *is* time to go further. This brings up the next *KEY* clinical point:

■ Question #2- *Is the QRS complex truly narrow?*

It is easy to get fooled ! Although it certainly *appears* that the QRS complex of the rhythm in Figure 1C-3 is narrow- one can *not* rule out the possibility that a portion of the QRS complex in this *single* monitoring lead might be lying *isoelectric* on the baseline:

- Obtaining a **12-lead ECG** while the patient is *still in* the tachycardia would help to confirm that the QRS complex is *truly* narrow in all 12 leads (and that the rhythm is *truly* supraventricular). Obtaining a 12-lead ECG during the tachycardia may also provide *diagnostic* assistance in determining the true mechanism of the arrhythmia, which may be invaluable for optimizing treatment.

- A 12-lead ECG should *not* be obtained if the patient is unstable. As emphasized, the treatment of choice for an unstable patient with tachycardia is *immediate* synchronized cardioversion- *regardless* of what the rhythm happens to be.

The *KEY* for deciding on optimal treatment of the various types of SVT lies with determining the **specific diagnosis** of the rhythm. This reflects the intent of our third clinical point:

- Question #3- *Is the diagnosis truly PSVT?*

As already discussed (in the section on *Differential Diagnosis*)- attention to parameters such as rate, regularity, and the presence and nature of atrial activity usually provides the clues that are needed for accurate diagnosis. Use of a vagal maneuver (*See below*) may provide additional assistance. For example, the narrow complex tachycardia in Figure 1C-3 is regular at a rate of approximately 180 beats/minute. Regularity of this rhythm rules out A Fib as a possibility. The heart rate of 180 beats/minute is too fast to be sinus tachycardia- and *not* consistent with that expected if the rhythm was A Flutter. This leaves **PSVT** as the *most likely* diagnosis. Initiation of treatment based on this presumptive diagnosis would now be in order.

Use of a Vagal Maneuver

Vagal maneuvers act by *transiently* increasing parasympathetic tone. This slows conduction through supraventricular and AV nodal tissues. One hopes to delay AV nodal conduction *just long enough* to interrupt the reentry circuit of PSVT and terminate the arrhythmia.

- In an emergency care setting- **cartotid sinus massage (CSM)** is the vagal maneuver performed most often for treatment. *Under constant ECG monitoring-* the patient's head is turned to the left and the area of the *right* carotid bifurcation (near the angle of the jaw) is gently but *firmly* massaged for 3-5 seconds at a time. If right carotid massage is ineffective, the left side may be tried. (One should *never* massage both sides simultaneously!)

- If PSVT persists despite application of a vagal maneuver- keep in mind that the maneuver may sometimes work if *reapplied* again *after* administration of antiarrhythmic therapy (since the effect of drugs and the maneuver are often synergistic).

■ In addition to its role in treatment, CSM may also be helpful as a ***diagnostic* maneuver** for distinguishing between the various types of SVT. When CSM is applied to a patient in PSVT- the rhythm will either be converted by the maneuver, or nothing will happen. In contrast, with sinus tachycardia or A Flutter-*transient* slowing of the ventricular response during massage will often allow "telltale" atrial activity to become apparent.

Note- CSM is *not* a totally benign maneuver-especially when applied to older individuals. Complications that have been associated with CSM include syncope, stroke, sinus arrest, high-grade AV block, prolonged asystole, and ventricular tachyarrhythmias in patients with digitalis intoxication. As a result- CSM should probaly *not* be attempted in patients with a history of sick sinus syndrome, cervical bruits, or cerebrovascular disease, or when the possibility of Digoxin toxicity exists.

Medical Therapy: *Adenosine and Verapamil*

The two drugs most commonly used for treatment of PSVT are Adenosine and Verapamil. Although AHA Guidelines now favor Adenosine as the drug of first choice for emergency treatment of this arrhythmia- we believe *both* drugs still retain a definite role in therapy.

■ *Adenosine*. The most remarkable pharmacologic feature of Adenosine relates to its rapid onset of action and exceedingly short half-life (which is estimated to be *less* than 10 seconds in duration!). A decided advantage of this feature is that the clinician will know within a very short period of time whether or not the drug will work. Side effects such as cough, flushing, and excessive bradycardia may occur- but even if they do, they are likely to be extremely short-lived.

- The recommended *initial* dose of Adenosine is to administer **6 mg** by **IV push**. If there is no response after 1-2 minutes- a 2nd dose (of **12**

mg) may be tried- and repeated (if needed) after another 1-2 minutes (for a *total* dose of 6 + 12 + 12 = **30 mg**). If this amount is ineffective, it is unlikely that Adenosine will work- and *alternative* therapy (i.e., IV Verapamil or Diltiazem) should be tried.

- Adenosine is one of the few drugs that *must* be given by **"IV push"**- injecting the drug *as fast as possible* (i.e., over a period of 1-3 seconds!). Failure to do so may result in the drug breaking down while still in the IV tubing. Drug distribution and absorption may be further facilitated by *immediately* following each dose with a **saline flush** (of ≈20 ml of fluid).

- The principal drawbacks of Adenosine are that the drug is ineffective for treatment of other types of SVT that are not dependent on AV nodal reentry (since slowing of the ventricular response with A Fib and A Flutter is so transient)- and that *recurrence* of PSVT is likely to occur in many patients after the effect of the drug wears off.

- **Verapamil.** Up until recently, Verapamil had been the pharmacologic agent of choice for emergency treatment of PSVT. When used appropriately, the drug is usually well tolerated and effective in converting this reentry tachyarrhythmia in more than 90% of cases. Additional advantages of Verapamil include the duration of action of its antiarrhythmic effect (which lasts for up to 30 minutes), availability of an oral formulation of the drug (which facilitates long-term antiarrhythmic control), and its efficacy in treating other types of SVT (including MAT, A Fib, and A Flutter). In contrast- Adenosine has a much shorter duration of action, is not available in an oral formulation, and is only effective in treatment of *reentry* tachyarrhythmias.

> **Note**- Clinical indications, cautions, and adverse effects that we list below for Verapamil are similar for Diltiazem. AHA Guidelines still favor use of IV Verapamil for treatment of PSVT- probably because of greater clinical experience accumulated with this drug (AHA Text- Pg 7-11).

- Dosing considerations for use of Verapamil in the treatment of PSVT are similar to those presented earlier in discussion of A Fib/ Flutter. Thus, **2.5-5 mg IV** may be given for the first dose of Verapamil- which may then be increased (to 5-10 mg) for a second IV dose given 15-30 minutes later (if/as needed).

- *Pretreatment* with IV infusion of **Calcium Chloride** (infusing 500-1,000 mg over a 5-10 minute period) has been shown to minimize the hypotensive response of Verapamil (or Diltiazem)- *without* diminishing drug efficacy for converting or controlling the ventricular response to supraventricular tachyarrhythmias. Such pretreatment might be considered particularly for patients with borderline hemodynamic status (i.e., systolic blood pressure of *less* than 100 mm Hg).

- The major concern regarding Verapamil (and Diltiazem) is to be sure that these drugs are *never* given to a patient who might have VT. If this were to happen, the vasodilatory and negative inotropic effects of these drugs would be likely to precipitate deterioration of the rhythm to V Fib. Verapamil (and Diltiazem) should therefore *never* be used as a diagnostic/therapeutic trial for treatment of a *wide-complex* tachycardia if the etiology of the rhythm is at all uncertain.

- A decided advantage of Verapamil (and Diltiazem) is that if IV use is successful in converting the rhythm- antiarrhythmic effect can then be maintained (and the chance of recurrence minimized) by continuing the patient on oral therapy.

Other Treatment Options

In almost all cases, use of either a vagal maneuver and/or treatment with Adenosine or Verapamil will be effective in converting the patient with PSVT to sinus rhythm. If it is not- other therapeutic options might be considered. These include:

- **Sedation**. Although not usually thought of as antiarrhythmic therapy- judicious use of a short-acting benzodiazepine (i.e., 0.5-1 mg of Ativan)- may produce a beneficial effect on the mechanism of PSVT. This is because the degree of autonomic tone at any given moment will directly influence conduction properties in AV nodal reentry pathways. As a result, in addition to relieving the anxiety that so often accompanies PSVT- use of sedation may produce a beneficial *physiologic* effect that significantly contributes to converting the arrhythmia.

- **Digoxin**. Although frequently used in the past to treat PSVT, the tremendous success of Adenosine and Verapamil have dramatically reduced current use of this drug for this indication. Thus despite the fact that Digoxin is effective for treating PSVT (and is still often used in long-term therapy)- the relatively delayed onset of action of this drug make it a *second-line* agent for treatment of PSVT in the emergency situation.

- **IV Beta-Blockers**. As is the case for the treatment of rapid A Fib/Flutter, IV beta-blockers seem to be used much less often than Adenosine or Verapamil for emergency treatment of PSVT. The reason for this is *not* a reflection of drug efficacy, since IV beta-blockers demonstrate comparable success rates for converting PSVT to sinus rhythm. Instead, it is probably because Adenosine is simpler (and perhaps safer) to use than IV beta-blockers- and because most emergency care providers are more comfortable with its use. As a result, Adenosine is usually tried first in the acute treatment protocol. If PSVT persists- IV Verapamil is usually tried next, which essentially precludes subsequent trial of an IV beta-blocker. Because of a cumulative AV nodal blocking effect, IV

Verapamil/Diltiazem and IV beta-blockers should *never* be given in close proximity (i.e., within 20-30 minutes) of each other- as the combination of these agents could lead to *marked* bradycardia (and even asystole!).

■ *Synchronized Cardioversion.* Because of the extremely high success rate of medical therapy for treatment of PSVT- synchronized cardioversion is *rarely* needed for treatment of this arrhythmia. In the rare event that it is needed, AHA Guidelines suggest *initial* use of **100 joules** for PSVT- increasing to 200, 300, and 360 joules as needed.

> **Note-** As is the case for treatment of other tachyarrhythmias, immediate synchronized cardioversion is indicated if hemodynamic instability develops *at any time* during the treatment process. Clinically, this is a relatively uncommon occurrence with PSVT.

■ *Diltiazem.* Although AHA Guidelines recommend Verapamil as the drug of second choice for medical treatment of PSVT- use of Diltiazem would seem to provide an equally effective alternative. When dosed appropriately, potential advantages of IV Diltiazem are less myocardial depression and a lower incidence of severe hypotension.

Dosing considerations for IV Diltiazem in the treatment of PSVT are similar to those presented earlier for IV bolus treatment of A Fib/ Flutter. Thus, an *initial* IV bolus of 0.25 mg/kg (which for an *average-sized* adult is ≈**15-20 mg**) is recommended- which may then be increased to 0.35 mg/kg (or about **25 mg**) for the second IV bolus that is given 15 minutes later if there is no response. Continuous IV infusion is rarely needed- since once the reentry cycle in PSVT is broken, the arrhythmia will be terminated. Recurrence may be prevented with long-term oral therapy.

Figure 1C-4- *Treatment Algorithm for VT*

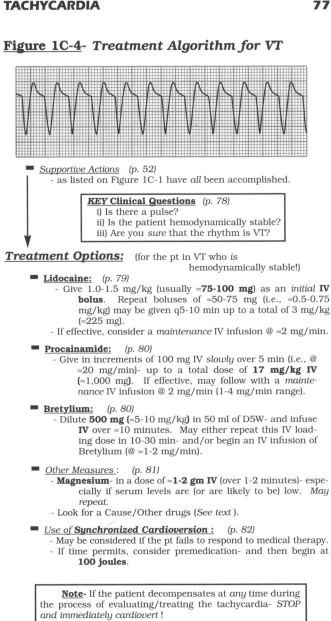

▬ *Supportive Actions*   (p. 52)
   - as listed on Figure 1C-1 have *all* been accomplished.

> **_KEY_ Clinical Questions**   (p. 78)
> i) Is there a pulse?
> ii) Is the patient hemodynamically stable?
> iii) Are you *sure* that the rhythm is VT?

Treatment Options: (for the pt in VT who *is*
                                          hemodynamically stable!)

▬ **Lidocaine:**   (p. 79)
   - Give 1.0-1.5 mg/kg (usually ≈**75-100 mg**) as an *initial* **IV bolus**.   Repeat boluses of ≈50-75 mg (i.e., ≈0.5-0.75 mg/kg) may be given q5-10 min up to a total of 3 mg/kg (≈225 mg).
   - If effective, consider a *maintenance* IV infusion @ ≈2 mg/min.

▬ **Procainamide:**   (p. 80)
   - Give in increments of 100 mg IV *slowly* over 5 min (i.e., @ ≈20 mg/min)- up to a total dose of **17 mg/kg IV** (≈1,000 mg).   If effective, may follow with a *maintenance* IV infusion @ 2 mg/min (1-4 mg/min range).

▬ **Bretylium:**   (p. 80)
   - Dilute **500 mg** (≈5-10 mg/kg) in 50 ml of D5W- and infuse **IV** over ≈10 minutes.   May either repeat this IV loading dose in 10-30 min- and/or begin an IV infusion of Bretylium (@ ≈1-2 mg/min).

▬ *Other Measures* :   (p. 81)
   - **Magnesium**- in a dose of ≈**1-2 gm IV** (over 1-2 minutes)- especially if serum levels are (or are likely to be) low.   *May repeat.*
   - Look for a Cause/Other drugs (*See text*).

▬ *Use of **Synchronized Cardioversion** :*   (p. 82)
   - May be considered if the pt fails to respond to medical therapy.
   - If time permits, consider premedication- and then begin at **100 joules**.

> **Note**- If the patient decompensates at *any* time during the process of evaluating/treating the tachycardia- *STOP and immediately cardiovert* !

Treatment Algorithm for Ventricular Tachycardia

AHA recommendations for emergency treatment of **sustained ventricular tachycardia (VT)** are summarized in the algorithm we present in <u>Figure 1C-4</u>. Assessment of the patient in *sustained* VT and selection of the optimal course of treatment for this arrhythmia are among the most problematic (and anxiety producing) tasks in emergency cardiac care. In the hope of facilitating the decision making process- we insert three *KEY Clinical Questions* into the earliest part of our approach.

Initial Approach: *KEY Clinical Questions*

Optimal management of sustained VT is best determined by *immediate* consideration of the following three questions:

> i) Is there a pulse?
> ii) Is the patient hemodynamically stable?
> iii) Are you *sure* that the rhythm is VT?

The purpose of these three questions is to hone in on the clinical significance of the arrhythmia, as well as to attempt to confirm the diagnosis. Clinical application of this *Initial Approach* can be illustrated by considering the rhythm shown at the top of Figure 1C-4. Clearly, the *most* important issue to address when confronted with a patient in a rhythm such as this is contained in the first question that we list above- **Is there a PULSE?** If the patient does *not* have a pulse, then the approach to the rhythm is simple- shock (*unsynchronized*) as soon as possible. As emphasized in Section 1B (*See Figure 1B-1*)- **Pulseless VT should be treated as V Fib** (i.e., with immediate *unsynchronized* defibrillation).

Approach to VT: *If a Pulse IS Present*

The approach to management of VT is significantly different when a pulse *IS* present. Highest priority is now given to determining the patient's hemodynamic status. There are two possibilities:

> i) *The patient may be* **hemodynamically UNSTABLE**- in which case the need for immediate action is urgent. As emphasized at the beginning of this section (and illustrated in Figure 1C-1 on page 51)- *immediate* synchronized cardioversion is indicated if serious signs and/or symptoms are being produced as a *direct result* of the tachycardia.

ii) *The patient may be* **hemodynamically STABLE**- in which case there should be (by definition) a little more time to reflect on the process. Ideally, the third clinical question can now be addressed and hopefully answered (i.e., **Are you sure that the rhythm is VT?**). If there is reasonable certainty of the clinical diagnosis- then a trial of medical therapy can be undertaken.

Hemodynamically Stable VT: *Medical Therapy*

Therapeutic options to consider in the management of hemodynamically stable VT are listed in Figure 1C-4. They include the following:

- **Lidocaine**. Lidocaine is generally accepted as the antiarrhythmic agent of choice for medical treatment of sustained VT. AHA Guidelines recommend a dose of 1.0-1.5 mg/kg (usually ≈**75-100 mg**) to be given as an *initial* **IV bolus**. Additional 50-75 mg IV boluses may follow every 5-10 minutes thereafter (either as needed- and/or until a *total* loading dose of *up to* 225 mg has been given). If Lidocaine appears to be effective- then a **maintenance IV infusion** (at a rate of **2 mg/minute**) should be started.

    - Although many clinicians tend to increase the Lidocaine infusion rate with each additional bolus of the drug that is given- this is *not* essential during the period of Lidocaine loading. On the contrary, routinely increasing the infusion rate (i.e., to 3 and 4 mg/minute) after administration of each Lidocaine bolus may *unnecessarily* increase the risk of developing Lidocaine toxicity. IV infusion at a rate of 2 mg/minute will be adequate for most patients.

    - On the other hand, if the ventricular arrhythmia rapidly resolves after bolus administration- only to recur *after* steady state conditions have been achieved (i.e., at an infusion rate of 2 mg/minute)- then administration of an *additional* 50 mg bolus of Lidocaine *and* an increase in the infusion rate (i.e., to 3 mg/minute) may be warranted.

- **Procainamide**.   If Lidocaine is ineffective- then Procainamide is generally recommended as the *second-line* agent of choice for medical treatment of sustained VT. The drug is most often given in **IV increments** of **100 mg** (administering each increment *slowly* over a 5 minute period)- until one of the following **end points** is achieved:

    > i) The patient receives an adequate loading dose. Although a loading dose of ≈500-1,000 mg is usually given, a total dose of *up to* **17 mg/kg IV** may be administered.
    >
    > ii) The arrhythmia is suppressed.
    >
    > iii) Hypotension develops.
    >
    > iv) QRS widening occurs.

    Alternatively, 500-1,000 mg of Procainamide may be diluted in 100 ml of D5W and administered as a loading IV infusion over 30-60 minutes.

    An additional advantage of using Procainamide is that even if the drug is not successful in converting the rhythm- it may still *slow* the ventricular response of VT (which may allow the patient to remain hemodynamically stable for a longer period of time).

> **Note**- If either loading regimen of Procainamide achieves the desired clinical effect- a continuous **IV** *maintenance* **infusion** of the drug may be started at a rate of **2 mg/minute** (range = 1-4 mg/minute).

- **Bretylium**.   Use of Bretylium for the treatment of VT has been deemphasized. Practically speaking, the drug appears to be much more effective as an *antifibrillatory* agent for use in refractory V Fib- than as an *antiarrhythmic* agent for the treatment of PVCs or VT. Moreover, the most common long-term adverse effect associated with Bretylium therapy is hypotension, which further limits its use. As a result, other therapeutic options could be considered if Lidocaine and Procainamide are ineffective (*See below*).

- If Bretylium is used for treatment of sustained VT- the drug should be given as an **IV loading infusion** rather than as bolus therapy. To do this, one ampule of Bretylium (= **500 mg**) is mixed in 50 ml of D5W- and then infused over a 10 minute period.

- Following IV loading, a **maintenance IV infusion** (at a rate of between **1-2 mg/minute**) may be started to sustain the drug's antiarrhythmic effect.

■ **Magnesium.** The role of Magnesium Sulfate in the treatment of *sustained* VT and cardiac arrest is still not clarified. As a result, use of the drug in this setting is still largely empiric.

- Consider IV Magnesium if the patient fails to respond to standard therapy- especially if hypomagnesemia is likely.

- The usual *initial* dose of Magnesium for VT is **1-2 gm IV**. If needed, this amount may be repeated. For life-threatening situations the drug can be administered over a 1-2 minute period. Slower administration, or use of a continuous IV infusion is appropriate when the situation is less urgent.

■ **Other Measures.** Several alternative measures may be considered if the patient with *sustained* VT fails to respond to the above treatment:

- **Search for a potentially correctable cause.** Persistent VT may result from the presence of any of the same factors that predispose to persistence of refractory V Fib (*See pages 30-31*).

- *Use of an* **IV Beta-Blocker.** Although *not* usually considered as first-line agents in the treatment of most tachyarrhythmias- there clearly *are* times when *all* other treatment measures will fail (and *only* IV beta-blockers may save the patient). This is especially true when excessive *sympathetic* tone is likely to be operative as a cause of the sustained VT.

- *Consideration of **IV Sotalol** or **Amiodarone***. These drugs are *not* yet included in AHA Guidelines. Experience in the setting of sustained VT and cardiac arrest is still somewhat limited- although initial reports are favorable. Use of these drugs may become more common in the not too distant future.

- **Synchronized Cardioversion**. In the event that medical therapy (as outlined above) is unsuccessful in converting the patient out of *sustained* VT- cardioversion may be tried. If the patient shows no signs of hemodynamic compromise, this may be attempted under **"semi-elective"** conditions. This entails:

    i) Sedation of the patient (i.e., with IV Valium, Versed, or other agent).
    ii) Calling anesthesia to the bedside to assist with intubation if needed (so as to leave you free to concentrate on managing the arrhythmia).

    AHA Guidelines recommend use of the *Standard Sequence of Energy Levels* for synchronized cardioversion of VT. One should therefore *begin* with **100 joules**- and increase to 200, 300, and then 360 joules (if/as needed). An exception to this recommendation is for the patient with *polymorphic VT*- which often requires higher energy levels (of 200 joules or more) for successful cardioversion (AHA Text- Pg 1-35).

If the Patient *Becomes* Hemodynamically Unstable

If at *any* time during the process of evaluation or treatment the patient *becomes* hemodynamically unstable- STOP the process. In this situation- *synchronized* cardioversion should be *immediately* performed.

- The clinical definition of *hemodynamically "unstable"* varies greatly. The KEY defining premise of the term is that signs and/or symptoms must be produced in association with the rhythm as a *direct result* of the rapid rate.

- AHA Guidelines emphasize that even when the decision to cardiovert *"immediately"* has been made- that medical therapy (i.e., use of Lidocaine, Procainamide, etc.) may *still* be tried- *IF* these drugs are *immediately* available- provided that giving these drugs *does not* result in delay of cardioversion (AHA Text- Pg 1-35). *Clinical judgement is needed at the bedside.*

Cough Version

If a pulse is present and the patient is alert- consider the use of **cough version.** Whether the mechanism for cough version is improved coronary perfusion (from the increase in intrathoracic pressure generated by the cough), activation of the autonomic nervous system, or conversion of mechanical energy from the cough (into an electrical depolarization), is unknown. What has been shown is that the cough may effectively convert sustained VT to normal sinus rhythm in a surprising number of cases.

- In practice, cough version appears to be vastly underutilized. The technique should probably be the *first* intervention for treatment of the conscious patient who presents in sustained VT.

- In contrast to cough version, use of the *precordial thump* has been strongly deemphasized as a treatment modality for sustained VT. The problem with the thump is that even though the maneuver may occasionally convert VT to sinus rhythm- it is equally likely (if not more so) to convert this rhythm to V Fib, asystole, or pulseless idioventricular rhythm. Thus, if synchronized cardioversion is readily available, it would seem to be far preferable to delivery of 2-5 joules at a *random* (and possibly vulnerable) point in the cardiac cycle as is provided by the thump.

Figure 1C-5- *Treatment Algorithm for WCT of Uncertain Type*

(When the patient is hemodynamically stable)

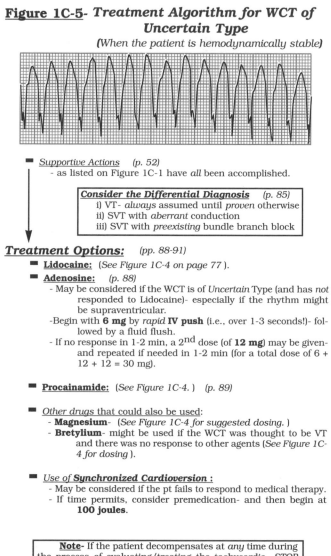

■ *Supportive Actions*   *(p. 52)*
  - as listed on Figure 1C-1 have *all* been accomplished.

> **Consider the Differential Diagnosis**   *(p. 85)*
> i) VT- *always* assumed until *proven* otherwise
> ii) SVT with *aberrant* conduction
> iii) SVT with *preexisting* bundle branch block

Treatment Options: *(pp. 88-91)*

■ **Lidocaine:**   *(See Figure 1C-4 on page 77).*

■ **Adenosine:**   *(p. 88)*
  - May be considered if the WCT is of *Uncertain* Type (and has *not* responded to Lidocaine)- especially if the rhythm might be supraventricular.
  -Begin with **6 mg** by *rapid* **IV push** (i.e., over 1-3 seconds!)- followed by a fluid flush.
  - If no response in 1-2 min, a 2nd dose (of **12 mg**) may be given- and repeated if needed in 1-2 min (for a total dose of 6 + 12 + 12 = 30 mg).

■ **Procainamide:**   *(See Figure 1C-4.)*   *(p. 89)*

■ *Other drugs* that could also be used:
  - **Magnesium**- *(See Figure 1C-4 for suggested dosing.)*
  - **Bretylium**- might be used if the WCT was thought to be VT and there was no response to other agents *(See Figure 1C-4 for dosing).*

■ *Use of* **Synchronized Cardioversion** :
  - May be considered if the pt fails to respond to medical therapy.
  - If time permits, consider premedication- and then begin at **100 joules**.

> **Note**- If the patient decompensates at *any* time during the process of evaluating/treating the tachycardia- *STOP and immediately cardiovert* !

Treatment Algorithm for WCT of *Uncertain* Type

AHA recommendations for emergency treatment of the patient with a **WCT** (**W**ide-**C**omplex **T**achycardia) of **Uncertain Type** are summarized in the algorithm we present in Figure 1C-5. In many ways, evaluation and management of this problem is similar to that for the patient with VT. The principal difference relates to the fact that *despite* QRS widening- the etiology of this rhythm is *not* quite as certain as it is for VT- hence use of the name, **WCT** of *"Uncertain" Type.* To facilitate the decision making process- the three major diagnostic considerations for WCT are incorporated into the initial part of our approach in this algorithm.

Differential Diagnosis of WCT: *Key Clinical Points*

For practical purposes, the differential diagnosis of a *WCT* of *Uncertain Type* consists of *three* major entities. They are:

      i) VT
      ii) SVT with *aberrant* conduction
      iii) SVT with *preexisting* bundle branch block

Detailed description of criteria used for distinguishing between VT and these two forms of SVT extends beyond the scope of this book. Nevertheless, the following *KEY* clinical points can be made about the approach we suggest for assessing the patient with **WCT** of **Uncertain** Type :

- **Until proven otherwise- always assume that the rhythm is VT.** Statistically, the etiology of a *WCT of Uncertain Type* is far more likely to be VT than SVT (with QRS widening from either aberrant conduction or preexisting bundle branch block). This dictum holds true *regardless* of whether the patient is alert or not- and *regardless* of what the blood pressure happens to be. **The patient should be treated accordingly** (i.e., as if the rhythm was VT- *until proven otherwise*).

- As was the case for evaluating the patient with VT (Figure 1C-4)- the *most* important question to address is the following: **Is the patient is hemodynamically stable**. If not- specific diagnosis of the tachyarrhythmia *no longer matters* (since *immediate* cardioversion should now be performed *regardless* of what the arrhythmia happens to be!).

- *If the patient IS hemodynamically* **STABLE**- then there may be time to evaluate the situation in more detail. Selecting the *most* appropriate therapeutic option for the patient with WCT of *Uncertain* Type will become *far* simpler if the correct diagnosis can be made- at least with *relative* certainty. Clues that may help in this regard (i.e., to distinguish between the three major causes of WCT) include one or more of the following:

    - *Recall of "the facts"*. Given that the overwhelming majority of WCTs of *Uncertain* Type will turn out to be VT- the onus must reside on proving that the rhythm is *not* VT- *and not the other way around.*

    - *Brief review of the patient's medical history*. Statistical odds that a regular WCT of *Uncertain* Type is VT approach 90% (!!!)- *IF* the patient in question is an ***older adult*** (i.e., >60-70 years old) *and* has a history of *documented* **heart disease** (i.e., *either* previous infarction, angina, or heart failure).

    - *Use of prior tracings*. A glance through the patient's medical chart to look for prior 12-lead ECGs and/or recent telemetry recordings may sometimes provide invaluable information. Prior tracings may reveal the longterm presence of *preexisting* bundle branch block, or WPW on a baseline ECG. Recent telemetry tracings may reveal other episodes of tachycardia that were *definitely* diagnosed to be VT, A Fib/Flutter, or MAT- and/or PVCs that manifest an *identical* morphologic appearance to that of the QRS complexes in the WCT being assessed.

- *Obtaining a **12-lead ECG** during the WCT*. If at all feasible, a 12-lead ECG should be obtained while the patient is still in the tachycardia. Atrial activity that might not be evident on a single lead recording may sometimes become *instantly* obvious in other leads obtained as part of the 12-lead tracing. Similarly, *seemingly narrow* QRS complexes in a single monitoring lead may *in reality* be surprisingly wide (if part of the QRS complex in the lead being monitored happens to lie *isoelectric* to the baseline). Finally, use of a few *KEY* (and surprisingly *easy* to remember) clues relating to QRS axis and QRS morphology may dramatically increase the diagnostic reliability of the ECG for those informed/experienced emergency care providers attentive to these findings.

Bottom Line- Assessing the patient *always* comes first! The most important issue to address in evaluating *any* patient who presents with a *WCT of Uncertain Type* is hemodynamic status. Subsequent management depends on this assessment. A 12-lead ECG should *not* be obtained if the patient is acutely unstable. Instead- *immediate* cardioversion is indicated for the unstable patient.

The point to emphasize is that if the patient *is* hemodynamically stable- then optimal management can *only* be selected if the correct ECG diagnosis is known. Appropriate use of a 12-lead ECG obtained *during* the tachycardia will greatly facilitate this determination much of the time. Simply stated, when evaluating a WCT of *unknown* etiology- ***"12 leads are BETTER than one"***.

- *Trial of a diagnostic maneuver*. This may either be in the form of a **vagal maneuver** (such as carotid massage or Valsalva)- and/or with use of **Adenosine** (i.e., *"chemical Valsalva"*)- *IF* deemed appropriate as determined by assessment of the tracing and the patient's clinical condition!

Vagal maneuvers are most likely to be helpful in the differential diagnosis of *narrow-complex* tachyarrhythmias (such as A Flutter, rapid A Fib, and rapid sinus tachycardia). They may even be *curative* if the rhythm is PSVT. In contrast, they rarely affect VT. Performance of a vagal maneuver may therefore be helpful from a *diagnostic* (as well as *therapeutic*) standpoint- if applied to a patient with a WCT that might well be supraventricular.

KEY- Performance of a vagal maneuver is *not* completely benign. As a result, it should probably *not* be done if you strongly suspect that the patient is in VT. Similarly, because Adenosine is *not* a completely benign medication- we prefer *not* to administer this drug to patients with probable VT.

On the other hand- use of *either* a vagal maneuver *and/or* "chemical Valsalva" (with Adenosine) is perfectly appropriate and often of invaluable assistance for evaluating patients with WCT that is at least *somewhat likely* to be of supraventricular etiology.

Treatment Options for WCT

The drugs that are listed in Figure 1C-5 for treatment of a WCT of *Uncertain* Type are virtually the same as those listed in Figure 1C-4 for treatment of VT- with the *exception* of Adenosine. (*Dosing specifics for these drugs is also the same as shown in Figure 1C-4 on page 77*).

- **Lidocaine**. AHA Guidelines recommend Lidocaine as the drug of 1st choice for medical treatment of *both* VT and WCT of *Uncertain* Type. Their reason for doing so is to emphasize the point that the *most* common cause (*by far!*) of a WCT is VT- for which Lidocaine is the drug of choice.

- **Adenosine**. As noted above, AHA Guidelines suggest use of Adenosine as a *diagnostic/therapeutic* trial when the etiology of the WCT is *uncertain* and

Lidocaine has *not* been effective. The advantage of using Adenosine in this situation is that _IF_ the rhythm turns out to be supraventricular, administration of this drug will usually either *slow* the rate enough to allow correct diagnosis- or convert the rhythm (if the WCT is PSVT). With rare exceptions, Adenosine is unlikely to do anything if the rhythm turns out to be VT. Although use of this drug is *not* completely benign- most of the time administration of Adenosine will *not* be deleterious even if the drug is inadvertently given to a patient who is in VT (since the duration of its action is so short).

- The recommended *initial* dose of Adenosine is **6 mg** by rapid **IV push** (i.e., given over 1-3 seconds!). If there is no response after 1-2 minutes, a 2nd dose (of **12 mg**) may be tried- and repeated (if needed) after another 1-2 minutes (for a *total* dose of 6 + 12 + 12 = **30 mg**).

Note- Unlike Adenosine (which *may* be used in the treatment of a WCT of *Uncertain* Type)- Verapamil and Diltiazem should **never** be used as a diagnostic/therapeutic trial to treat WCT unless it is known *with certainty* that the rhythm is supraventricular. Empiric treatment of a WCT with Verapamil (or Diltiazem) could be a "lethal error" if the WCT turned out to be VT (AHA Text- Pg 1-38).

- **Procainamide**. AHA Guidelines recommend Procainamide as the 3rd drug to use in the treatment protocol for WCT- if Lidocaine and Adenosine have not been effective. An advantage of Procainamide over other antiarrhythmic agents is that this drug may be effective in treating a WCT- *regardless* of what the rhythm happens to be:

  - _If the WCT turns out to be VT_- Procainamide may either convert the rhythm- or at least slow down the rate of the VT.

  - _If the WCT turns out to be an SVT_- the "Quinidine-like" action of Procainamide may either convert the rhythm- and/or prevent recurrence (by suppressing PACs/PJCs that typically precipitate these tachyarrhythmias).

- *If the WCT turns out to be WPW*- Procainamide is the drug of choice for treatment of a WCT due to rapid A Fib in a patient with WPW. The reason Procainamide is effective for this indication is that it *slows* anterograde conduction down the accessory pathway. In contrast, Digoxin, Verapamil, and Diltiazem are all *contraindicated* for treatment of rapid A Fib with WPW because these drugs *accelerate* conduction in the forward direction down the accessory pathway.

Bottom Line- Regarding the approach we suggest to the patient with WCT of *Uncertain* Type:

- *Lidocaine* is clearly the drug of choice for *initial* treatment of a WCT that is thought to be VT. Statistically, this should be the most common situation encountered.

- *Adenosine* offers the advantage of effectiveness for treatment of PSVT- and diagnostic utility for determining the specific etiology of other types of SVT. We prefer *not* to give this drug if we think that the rhythm is really VT- but advocate its use if Lidocaine has been ineffective *and* an SVT appears to be more likely.

- *Procainamide* is a little bit more difficult to use than the other two drugs- but may help in treatment *regardless* of what the cause of the WCT happens to be.

- *Other Measures*. As was the case for VT, consideration might also be given to use of additional measures if the patient with sustained WCT fails to respond to Lidocaine/Adenosine/Procainamide. These may include:

  - *Search for a potentially correctable cause of the rhythm.*
  - *Use of **Magnesium**-* which may be helpful in the treatment of *both* VT and certain SVTs (especially when serum magnesium levels are likely to be low).

- *Use of **Bretylium**- which has become a 3rd-line agent for the treatment of sustained ventricular arrhythmias- but which may still be useful in selected cases.

- *Use of **Synchronized Cardioversion**. As was the case for VT, synchronized cardioversion should be considered if medical therapy (as outlined above) fails- and/or if at *any* time in the process the patient shows signs of hemodynamic compromise.

Questions to Further Understanding

What Should Be Done FIRST- If Your Patient is in a Sustained Tachycardia?

If your patient is in a *sustained* tachycardia:

   i) *DON'T* panic !!!
   ii) Remember to assess the patient in the manner suggested in Figure 1C-1 (on page 51).

The *KEY* to evaluation and management of *any* sustained tachycardia lies with first determing if a pulse is present. If not- then *immediate* countershock (i.e., *unsynchronized* defibrillation) is in order.

If a palpable pulse is present- it then becomes essential to determine whether or not the patient is hemodynamically stable. If the patient is unstable- *synchronized cardioversion* will take precedence over all other forms of therapy. On the other hand, if the patient in sustained tachycardia is hemodynamically stable- there is at least some time to attempt to determine the **specific diagnosis** of the rhythm- and then to follow with a trial of medical therapy based on this diagnosis.

How to determine Hemodynamic Stability in a Patient with Tachycardia?

As noted above, the most important parameter to assess in a patient with **tachycardia** is whether the rhythm is *hemodynamically* "significant". Specifically, the question to address is whether the rhythm is causing the patient problems (i.e., producing *signs* or *symptoms* of concern) as a *direct result* of the rate:

- **_Signs of Concern_**- include hypotension (i.e., systolic BP ≤80-90 mm Hg), shock, heart failure/pulmonary edema, and/or Acute MI.

- **_Symptoms of Concern_**- include chest pain, shortness of breath, and/or decreased mental status.

We emphasize that definition of **hemodynamic stability** is equally applicable for *SUPRAventricular* tachyarrhythmias- as it is for VT. Thus, a patient with tachycardia who is hypotensive, having chest pain, and mentally confused is probably in need of immediate cardioversion- *regardless* of whether the rhythm is VT or SVT. Additional points to keep in mind are:

i) that immediate cardioversion will usually *not* be needed when the heart rate of the tachycardia is *less than* 150 beats/minute (AHA Text- Pg 1-33).

ii) that some patients with sustained VT may be hemodynamically stable- and that they may *remain* in VT for surprisingly *long* periods of time (of minutes, hours- *and even days!*).

iii) that blood pressure determination can *not* be used as a discriminating factor to determine the etiology of the rhythm. Selected patients may even be *hypertensive* (with systolic BP readings that approach 200 mm Hg)- despite remaining in sustained VT for long periods of time.

iv) that bedside clinical evaluation (i.e., *"You have to be there"*) is usually the best way to determine the need for specific treatment. Thus, a patient in VT may not necessarily need immediate cardioversion *despite* a blood pressure reading of 70 systolic- _IF_ they are otherwise alert, comfortable, and asymptomatic.

v) that a patient does *not* necessarily need to be alert in order to be hemodynamically "stable". Many *other* factors may account for persistent lack of consciousness in the setting of cardiac arrest- including severe metabolic insult, residual effects from drug overdose, and a postictal state. Thus, *despite* continued unresponsiveness- a patient in a *sustained* tachycardia may remain *hemodynamically* stable for as long as the rhythm is associated with evidence of adequate perfusion (i.e., good peripheral pulses and an acceptable systolic blood pressure).

> **Note**- Keep in mind that virtually *identical* parameters are used to assess hemodynamic significance for a patient with **bradycardia**- as for *tachycardia* (i.e, the presence of associated hypotension, chest pain, shortness of breath, altered mental function, development of heart failure, etc.).

What If You are UNCERTAIN about the Etiology of the Rhythm?

An extremely important clinical entity in emergency cardiac care regards evaluation and management of the patient with a **WCT** (**W**ide-**C**omplex **T**achycardia) of **Uncertain** **Etiology**. Clinically we define this entity as the presence of a tachycardia in which the QRS complex is *wide* (i.e., ≥0.12 second)- and *normal* atrial activity is absent (or at least *not* immediately evident). In most cases, the ventricular rhythm will be regular (or at least *almost* regular)- although we emphasize that VT need *not* necessarily be a regular rhythm. Marked irregularity of the ventricular response (i.e., the presence of an *irregularly* irregular rhythm in which R-R intervals *continually* change from beat to beat)- suggests A Fib, in which QRS widening is likely to result from *preexisting* bundle branch block. Less marked irregularity of a WCT rhythm could represent *either* VT- or SVT (with aberrant conduction or bundle branch block).

The rhythm below is an example of a regular WCT (Figure 1C-6). The rate of this tachycardia is about 230 beats/minute, and there is no evidence of atrial activity.

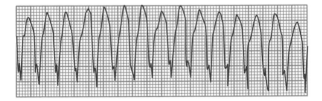

Figure 1C-6: *WCT of Uncertain Etiology.*

Clinically- the approach we suggest when confronted with a rhythm such as that shown in Figure 1C-6 consists of the following:

- *FIRST- Determine the patient's* **hemodynamic status**. As already emphasized, this is *by far* the most important action to accomplish. If the patient is hemodynamically unstable- *specific diagnosis* of the tachyarrhythmia *no longer matters*. This is because synchronized cardioversion now becomes *immediately* indicated *regardless* of what the rhythm happens to be.

- *IF the patient IS hemodynamically STABLE-* there may then be time to try to determine the etiology of the arrhythmia. This may be done by obtaining a **12-lead ECG** (*during* the tachycardia!)- and comparing it to prior 12-lead tracings or rhythm strips on the patient- and/or considering use of vagal maneuvers *if/as* appropriate. Remember that **sustained VT** is statistically far more likely to be the cause of a WCT than *SUPRAventricular* tachycardia with either aberrant conduction or preexisting bundle branch block. This is especially true if the WCT occurs in an *older* patient who has *underlying* heart disease.

- *IF doubt remains* (about the diagnosis): **Assume VT-** and **treat the patient accordingly!** This dictum holds true *regardless* of how stable the patient looks (and *regardless* of the patient's blood pressure).

- *Avoid* use of Verapamil/Diltiazem in the treatment of WCT (unless you are *100% certain* of a *SUPRAventricular* etiology).

- *Regarding specific treatment-* AHA Guidelines recommend trying **Lidocaine** first (on the assumption that the rhythm is most probably VT). This may be followed with **Adenosine** (if Lidocaine is unsuccessful)- and then **Procainamide**- and/or **Magnesium** (if deficiency of this cation is suspected)- and/or **Bretylium**. If hemodynamic decompensation occurs at *any* time during the process- prepare for *immediate* **synchronized cardioversion**. Cardioversion may also be appropriate when the patient fails to respond to medical therapy (AHA Text- Pg 1-33).

> **Note**- Keep in mind that Adenosine is likely to convert the rhythm *only* if the WCT is *supraventricular* with a mechanism of *reentry* (i.e., primarily PSVT). We therefore prefer *not* to use this drug if we strongly suspect VT as the etiology.

What If Medical Therapy of a Patient with Hemodynamically Stable VT is Ineffective?

If a patient with presumed VT fails to respond to a full trial of medical therapy (i.e., with Lidocaine, Procainamide, and other measures such as Bretylium, an IV ß-blocker, and/or Magnesium Sulfate)- then **synchronized cardioversion** may be in order.

- As long as a patient in sustained VT remains hemodynamically stable- synchronized cardioversion may be performed under *"semi-elective"* circumstances (i.e., with sedation and assistance from anesthesia).

- As already mentioned- if the possibility exists that the tachycardia being treated could be supraventricular (and not VT!)- then *empiric* administration of **Adenosine** is a reasonable therapeutic option.

Why is Cardioversion Safer than Unsynchronized Countershock?

The advantage of **synchronized** cardioversion is that the electrical discharge is programmed to occur on the upstroke of the R wave (i.e., at a point *away* from the "vulnerable period"). This greatly reduces the chance that the electrical impulse will occur at a time that precipitates deterioration of the rhythm to V Fib. In contrast with defibrillation, delivery of the electrical impulse is completely *unsynchronized*- and therefore equally likely to occur at any point in the cardiac cycle.

What if Synchronized Cardioversion Produces V Fib?

Although *synchronization* to the upstroke of the R wave minimizes the chance that the electrical impulse will be delivered during the "vulnerable period"- it does *not* eliminate this possibility. Thus despite the most appropriate of precautions- synchronized cardioversion may occasionally precipitate deterioration of a tachycardia to V Fib.

Comfort can at least be taken in the fact that even if V Fib is produced by cardioversion, the chance for converting the patient out of this rhythm is excellent. This is because you are right on the scene- and the time from recognition of this complication until action (i.e., defibrillation) should be minimal. *Anticipate this possibility.* Know that even if synchronized cardioversion precipitates development of V Fib- you will probably be able to save the patient by *immediately* deactivating the synchronizer mode and defibrillating the patient (with 200-360 joules). Modern defibrillators facilitate defibrillation in this situation because they *automatically* deactivate the synchronizer mode after electrical discharge.

What if the Cardioverter Won't Work?

There are numerous cardioverter/defibrillators on the market. Each features nuances in operation that distinguish one particular model from the next. In many hospitals, different types of defibrillators are present in different patient care areas. The point to emphasize is that the time to learn about operation of all of the various types of defibrillators that are used in your hospital is *not* in the middle of a code.

- If you do find yourself confronted with a patient in *sustained* VT who is in need of electrical therapy- and you are *unable* to get the defibrillator to deliver a synchronized impulse (for *whatever* reason) . . . . - do *not* spend more than a few moments trying to get the device to work. Instead, simply turn off the synchronizer switch- and *defibrillate* the patient.

- Delivery of an *unsynchronized* shock will successfully convert most cases of VT (albeit at a slightly increased risk compared to the use of synchronized cardioversion). The reason for not delaying defibrillation for more than a few moments is that delivery of an unsynchronized countershock to a hemodynamically unstable patient in VT is far preferable to delivery of no electrical energy at all.

What if the Rhythm is a Supraventricular Tachycardia?

The rhythm shown below (in <u>Figure 1C-7</u>) appears to be a ***regular SVT*** (**S**upra**V**entricular **T**achycardia) at a heart rate of about **220 beats/minute**. There is no clear evidence of atrial activity.

Lead II

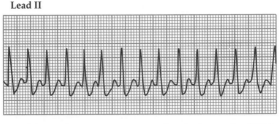

Figure 1C-7: Supraventricular Tachycardia (SVT).

The clinical problem is what to do when confronted with a rhythm such as that shown in Figure 1C-7- which is *presumed* to be an SVT. The approach we suggest consists of the following:

- *FIRST- Determine the patient's* **hemodynamic status**. This initial step is *equally* important when the rhythm is SVT- as it is when the rhythm is VT. This is because- *IF* the patient is acutely unstable, then *immediate* synchronized cardioversion is indicated *regardless* of what the rhythm happens to be.

- *IF the patient is hemodynamically STABLE*- then there is time to try to determine the etiology of the tachyarrhythmia. The *first* step in this process is to **verify that the rhythm is *truly* supraventricular**. *It is all too easy to get fooled*- because on occasion, a portion of the QRS complex may lie on the baseline. When this occurs- the QRS complex may look to be narrower than it really is. Thus, although the QRS complex in this particular case *appears* to be narrow- one can *not* be certain of this from inspection of the *single* monitoring lead shown above (i.e., it is hard to be sure in this tracing where the QRS complex ends- and the ST segment begins). Our clinical approach would clearly be different if the QRS complex was wide instead of narrow (which would make the rhythm a WCT of *uncertain* etiology).

> **Bottom Line**- If at all possible, it helps to obtain a *12-lead* **ECG** on the patient *during* the tachycardia. Doing so at the *earliest* feasible moment (i.e., assuming that the patient is hemo-dynamically stable)- may provide invaluable information:
> - it confirms that the QRS complex is *truly* narrow in all 12 leads (or that the QRS is wide)
> - it may reveal evidence of atrial activity that was not initially seen in the lead being monitored
> - it may provide additional information that helps in the diagnostic process.

■ *IF you confirm SVT and the patient is STABLE*- one should now proceed with **differential diagnosis**. Optimal treatment depends on determining the etiology of the SVT. Practically speaking- there are 3 clinical entities to consider in the differential diagnosis of a **regular SVT**. They are:

> i) Sinus Tachycardia
> ii) Atrial Flutter
> iii) PSVT.

Regularity of the rhythm *rules out* A Fib (although care should be taken in determining regularity- because *rapid* A Fib may *almost* look regular).

Distinction between the 3 entities listed above can often be made on the basis of clues provided by the 12-lead ECG (obtained *during* the tachycardia), by comparison of the tachycardia with prior tracings on the patient, and/or by use of a vagal maneuver (*See page 99*). All of these measures may help to reveal the nature of atrial activity (and/or the *lack* thereof).

KEY- We emphasize the importance of determining **heart rate** in the diagnostic process:

- **Sinus Tachycardia**- rarely exceeds 150-160 beats/minute in a supine (i.e., hospitalized) adult. A rate of 220 beats/minute (as is present in this case) is therefore clearly too fast to be sinus tachycardia.

- **Atrial Flutter**- almost always presents with a ventricular response that is close to 150 beats/minute (in the *untreated* patient). This is because the atrial rate of untreated flutter is almost always *close* to 300/minute (250-350 range)- and the AV node most commonly allows 2:1 AV conduction (i.e., 300 ÷ 2 ≈ 150 beats/minute).

    By the process of elimination- the rhythm in this case is most likely to be **PSVT** (since a rate of 220 beats/minute is highly unlikely for either sinus tachycardia or A Flutter).

- *Consider a **vagal maneuver***- as either a diagnostic and/or therapeutic trial. Application of a vagal maneuver will either abruptly convert PSVT to normal sinus rhythm- or have no effect at all. In contrast, if applied to a patient in sinus tachycardia, A Fib, or A Flutter- a vagal maneuver is likely to transiently *slow* the ventricular response (and in so doing hopefully allow recognition of the underlying atrial mechanism).

- *Begin drug therapy (based on your best guess of the etiology of the rhythm).* AHA Guidelines recommend **Adenosine** as the drug of 1st choice for the treatment of PSVT (AHA Text- Pg 1-33). If Adenosine is ineffective, consideration might then be given to the use of *Verapamil/Diltiazem.*

    AHA Guidelines also recommend Adenosine as the drug of 1st choice for treatment of SVT when the etiology is uncertain (AHA Text- Pg 1-33). Even if the drug fails to convert the rhythm- it is likely to *transiently* slow the rate enough to allow correct diagnosis (i.e., *"chemical Valsalva"*).

The optimal treatment approach differs slightly for the other forms of SVT. Rate-slowing drugs (i.e., Verapamil/Diltiazem, Digoxin, or beta-blockers) are often used first with rapid A Fib/Flutter. Conversion of these rhythms can then be achieved by correction of the underlying/pre-cipitating disorder, addition of other antiarrhythmic agents (i.e., Quinidine, Procainamide, etc.)- and/or synchronized cardioversion (if needed). A point to emphasize is that treatment of A Fib/Flutter may *not* necessarily be needed in the acute care setting if the ventricular response is not very rapid and the patient is hemodynamically stable.

The last diagnostic entity in the list- *sinus tachycardia*- is generally *not* treated with drugs. Instead, the treatment of choice for sinus tachycardia should always be aimed at identifying and correcting the underlying cause of this disorder.

Is it Likely that Adenosine will Replace Verapamil for the Treatment of PSVT? for Treatment of Other Arrhythmias?

No. Despite comparable efficacy for initial conversion rates of PSVT- individual characteristics of Adenosine and Verapamil are likely to preserve a separate niche for each of these agents.

- The principal advantages of **Adenosine** result from its *rapid* onset of action and ultra-short half-life. These features allow expeditious control of the arrhythmia in most cases. Adverse effects are usually of minimal clinical significance because they so rapidly resolve- and the drug is unlikely to be harmful if *inadvertently* given to a patient with a WCT that turns out to be VT.

- Administration of Adenosine may also be used as a *diagnostic* maneuver. Thus, the transient slowing of AV conduction produced by the drug may serve as a *"chemical Valsalva"* to facilitate identification of atrial activity that was not readily apparent on the initial tracing.

- The principal disadvantages of Adenosine are its cost and the high rate of PSVT recurrence after initial conversion to sinus rhythm. **Verapamil** is far more economical. The longer half-life of Verapamil's IV preparation lessens the chance of immediate recurrence- and availability of an oral formulation of Verapamil facilitates long-term antiarrhythmic control. Verapamil offers an additional advantage of efficacy for treatment of other supraventricular tachyarrhythmias (such as A Fib, A Flutter, and MAT). In contrast, Adenosine is unlikely to be effective for arrhythmias other than PSVT (i.e., it only *transiently* slows the ventricular response to A Fib/Flutter- and then the drug wears off).

> **Note-** A final point to consider is that although *both* Adenosine and Verapamil are more than 90% effective in the initial conversion of *reentry* tachyarrhythmias (such as PSVT)- these drugs *won't* always work. Failure to respond to one of these agents is an indication to try the other (which may then be successful!).

What are the Principal Points to Consider when Deciding whether to Use IV Verapamil or IV Diltiazem?

Clinical indications for using Verapamil are the *same* as for Diltiazem. Although the mechanism of action, cautions and adverse effects of these two drugs are also quite similar- there are some differences:

- IV Diltiazem appears to be somewhat *less* likely to produce hypotension and depression of left ventricular function than IV Verapamil (provided that *comparable* doses of each drug are used).

- Availability of an approved formulation for IV infusion of Diltiazem may further contribute to its safety by allowing *moment-to-moment* titration capability.

- Serum Digoxin levels seem to be affected to a much greater degree by concomitant use of Verapamil than they are by Diltiazem. With long-term use of Verapamil, the serum Digoxin level may *increase* by as much as 50%. In contrast, use of Diltiazem tends to increase serum Digoxin levels by only a small (and usually clinically unimportant) amount.

Note- The clinical niche for IV Diltiazem is probably in the management of *rapid* A Fib. The drug is highly effective in *slowing* the ventricular response to this rhythm, with an onset of action *within* 3 minutes of administering an IV bolus. Availability of a *continuous* IV infusion is a decided advantage of Diltiazem over Verapamil and Digoxin- and obviates having to continuously bolus the patient to control the rate.

What if in Treating SVT with IV Verapamil/Diltiazem the Patient Suddenly Develops Excessive Bradycardia or Asystole?

Despite awareness of all appropriate precautions- potentially serious adverse effects may still occur from acute administration of *either* IV Verapamil or IV Diltiazem. Manifestations of acute **Calcium Channel Blocker Toxicity** include profound brady-cardia, hypotension- and *even* asystole. AHA Guidelines recommend the following treatment approach to this problem (AHA Text- Pg 10-23):

i) If not done already- immediately *stop* administration of IV Verapamil/Diltiazem.

ii) Treat hypotension with fluid administration- rapidly giving 500-1,000 ml of **Normal Saline.**

iii) If there is no response to Saline- give **Calcium Chloride** (500-1,000 mg)- which may be repeated one or more times (up to a maximal dose of 2-4 g).

iv) Give **Epinephrine** (by IV bolus or IV infusion- depending on the rhythm). Keep in mind that in *refractory* cases- Epinephrine may *sensitize* the vasculature to the action of calcium. Therefore, be sure to *repeat* the Calcium Chloride dose *after* giving Epinephrine if the patient still has not responded.

v) Consider the use of **Glucagon** (in a dose of 1 to 5 mg IV).
vi) Consider *pacing.*
vii) Consider the use of *other* pressor agents *in addition* to
Epinephrine (i.e, Dopamine, Norepinephrine).

Note- Although it should seem intuitively obvious to treat *Calcium Channel Blocker Toxicity* with
Calcium Chloride- use of this drug is often *over-
looked* in this situation.   *Don't forget Calcium
Chloride.*

Atropine may be tried- but this drug is generally *not* very effective for the treatment of bradycardia caused by calcium channel blocker toxicity.

What if the Tachycardia being treated is Torsade de Pointes?

Management of the patient will be significantly different if
the rhythm being treated is **Torsade de Pointes**- than if the
rhythm is VT or WCT of *uncertain* etiology (Figure 1C-8).

Lead II

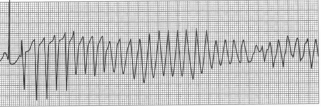

Figure 1C-8: Torsade de Pointes

The term *Torsade de Pointes* means *"twisting of the points".*
As can be seen from the example shown above, the term was
selected to reflect *alternating polarity* (i.e., from positive to negative) of the QRS complex with respect to the ECG baseline.
Diagnostically- *Torsade* is differentiated from "typical" (i.e.,
monophasic) VT by marked variation in QRS morphology *during*
the tachycardia.

Torsade is often asssociated with preexisting **QT prolonga-tion**. Early recognition of this rhythm is extremely important-because treatment differs greatly from that of "conventional" VT. The clinical approach we suggest to Torsade is as follows:

- *FIRST*- Determine the patient's hemodynamic status. **Cardiovert** (or **defibrillate**) the patient if acutely unstable. Although often responsive to electrical therapy- Torsade has the disturbing tendency to *repeatedly* recur (often until the underlying *cause* of the rhythm can be found and corrected).

- *As soon as possible*- Identify and treat the underlying cause of the rhythm. Common precipitating causes of *Torsade* to consider include overdose with tricyclic antidepressants or phenothiaziness, hypoka-lemia/hypomagnesemia, and/or use of drugs that lengthen the QT (such as Quinidine or Procainamide). Be sure to *avoid* use of IV Pro-cainamide when treating a patient with Torsade!

- Give **Magnesium Sulfate-** in a dose of **1-2 gm IV** (over 1-2 minutes)- which may be repeated one or more times. AHA Guidelines indicate that *higher* doses of Magnesium (i.e., of up to 5-10 gm) have been used with success in the treatment of some patients with Torsade (AHA Text- Pg 1-39).

- If Magnesium is ineffective- consider **overdrive pacing** (if available) as the next treatment of choice.

Bradyarrhythmias
(including PEA/Asystole)

The bradyarrhythmias encompass a wide variety of rhythm disturbances that range from the most often innocent *sinus bradycardia-* to the almost invariably lethal pulseless rhythms of *asystole* and *PEA*. Prognosis and recommendations for management depend on the particular rhythm itself, the associated clinical setting, and the patient's hemodynamic status.

- Definition. The term **"bradycardia"** technically refers to rhythms in which the heart rate is *below* **60 beats/minute**. AHA Guidelines simplify classification of these rhythms by defining them as that group of rhythms for which the heart rate is said to be **"too SLOW"**

> **Note-** An additional term- **"relative bradycardia"** - is used to refer to those rhythms that are faster than 60 beats/minute- but still *inappropriately SLOW* for the clinical situation at hand. For example, a patient in shock should normally develop a tachycardia to compensate for the drop in blood pressure. Although a heart rate of 70 beats/minute would *not* technically qualify as "bradycardia" in such a patient- this rate is still *inappropriately* slow (i.e., a *"relative"* bradycardia)- given the clinical setting of shock and marked hypotension.

- Other Bradyarrhythmias- Asystole and PEA are included in this section because principles for evaluation and treatment of these rhythms are essentially the same as those that are used for the other bradyarrhythmias.

Pulseless Electrical Activity

The term **PEA** (**P**ulseless **E**lectrical **A**ctivity) has been added to AHA Guidelines in an attempt to *unify* an otherwise complex group of cardiac rhythms. Similarities among the entities included in this group are that they all share a common list of potential etiologies- and that they generally respond to the same treatment protocol. Encompassed by this newer term are many rhythms that had previously been designated as *EMD* (*ElectroMechanical Dissociation*).

Clinically, the meaning of the term PEA is suggested by its name. Thus, the term is used to describe a group of diverse electrocardiographic rhythms that *by definition* manifest evidence of *Electrical Activity* (since they all produce an ECG rhythm)- but which are unified by the clinical finding of *Pulselessness*. According to this definition, PEA rhythms must therefore be *non-perfusing*- or at most no more than *minimally* perfusing (since they are by definition associated with the pulseless state).

Many types of ECG rhythms have been associated with the clinical entity known as PEA. Most can be classified into one of the following groups:

- **EMD Rhythms**- in which there is an *organized* ECG rhythm (usually with a *narrow* QRS complex)- but no pulse.

- **Pseudo-EMD Rhythms**- in which the ECG rhythm is associated with at least some *meaningful* mechanical contraction (as might be evidenced by obtaining a pulse with doppler that is too faint to palpate clinically).

- **Idioventricular** or **Ventricular Escape Rhythms**- in which the QRS complex of the escape rhythm is widened. Atrial activity is absent. There is no pulse. Included in this group are *post-defibrillation* idioventricular rhythms.

- **Bradyasystolic Rhythms**- in which there is profound bradycardia, often with prolonged periods of asystole. There is no pulse.

An essential point to emphasize about PEA rhythms is that they are often associated with *specific* clinical states that *can* be reversed- *IF* these states can be *identified early* and *treated appropriately* (AHA Text- Pg 1-21).

> **Note**- The ECG appearance of a PEA rhythm
> may provide insight as to the relative likelihood that
> the condition can be reversed. In general, progno-
> sis tends to be better if the ECG rhythm manifests
> *organized* atrial activity (in the form of P waves that
> conduct), a rate that is *not* excessively slow, and
> *narrow* QRS complexes.
>   In contrast- PEA is much more likely to be a
> *preterminal* rhythm when organized atrial activity is
> absent, the QRS complex is wide, and/or bradycar-
> dia persists despite medical treatment.

Treatment Algorithm for PEA Rhythms

AHA recommendations for treatment of the **PEA rhythms**
are summarized in the algorithm we present in Figure 1D-1.
Management priorities are best understood by awareness of the
following two *KEY* clinical points:

i) That by definition- **PEA is a *nonperfusing*** (or at least *not
adequately* perfusing) **rhythm**.
ii) That PEA is almost always a **secondary disorder** (that
occurs as a result of *some other* underlying condition).

KEY Treatment Options : CPR/Epinephrine

Because PEA is a *non-perfusing* (or at most a *minimally* perfusing) rhythm- the *initial* priority in management must logically
be to **begin CPR** (and/or to **continue CPR** if it has already been
started). CPR will need to be performed for as long as the patient
remains pulseless.

The medical treatment of choice for PEA is **Epinephrine.**
Use of this drug increases aortic diastolic pressure and prefer-
entially shunts blood from the external to the internal carotid
artery- actions which favor the maintenance of blood flow to the
heart and the brain. Epinephrine also exerts a potent inotropic
and chronotropic effect (to increase the force and rate of contraction).

- Epinephrine may be given either *intravenously* (**IV**) or
endotracheally (**ET**)- depending on whichever route of
access is established first. Although IV administration is preferable- do *not* hesitate to use the ET route

if this is the only access available for drug delivery. A larger dose (i.e., **2-2.5 mg**) should be used when giving Epinephrine by the ***ET route***.

■ If adequate IV access is available- the *initial* recommended dose of **Epinephrine** for treatment of PEA is **1.0 mg IV** (or 10 ml of a 1:10,000 soln.). This amount of drug is referred to as an **SDE** dose (i.e., **S**tandard-**D**ose **E**pinephrine).

■ The effect of an IV bolus of Epinephrine peaks in about 2-3 minutes. As a result, the drug should probably be repeated *at least* every 3-5 minutes- for as long as the PEA rhythm persists.

■ During cardiac arrest- AHA Guidelines allow for *flexibility* in Epinephrine dosing if the patient fails to respond to the initial SDE dose (AHA Text- Pg 1-16). One may therefore *either* repeat the 1 mg SDE dose in 3-5 minutes (and continue thereafter as needed with 1 mg doses)- **or** *choose between several* **H**igh-**D**ose **alternative** *regimens.* These include:

    i) Administration of **2-5 mg** IV boluses (which AHA Guidelines describe as *"intermediate"* dose Epinephrine)

    - OR -

    ii) *Escalating* **1- 3- 5 mg** IV boluses

    - OR -

    iii) Dosing at **0.1 mg/kg** as an IV bolus.

Note- Lower doses of Epinephrine (i.e., SDE) are more likely to work for the subgroup of patients with less severe forms of PEA. Such patients probably have at least some meaningful contractile actvity (which is why they may be more likely to respond to therapy). Clinical features that help to identify such individuals include detection of a pulse by doppler, a higher initial ET CO_2 reading- and/or ECG findings of an organized rhythm with conducting P waves and narrow QRS complexes.

In contrast- SDE dosing would seem to be less likely to work when there is no contractile activity (as suggested when no pulse is detected by doppler, the initial ET CO_2 reading is low, and a wide QRS complex rhythm is present that is slow and lacks P waves). Higher doses of Epinephrine should probably be considered at an *earlier* point for such individuals (if they are felt to be salvageable)- and even then, realistic chances for long-term survival are poor.

Figure 1D-1- *Treatment Algorithm for PEA*

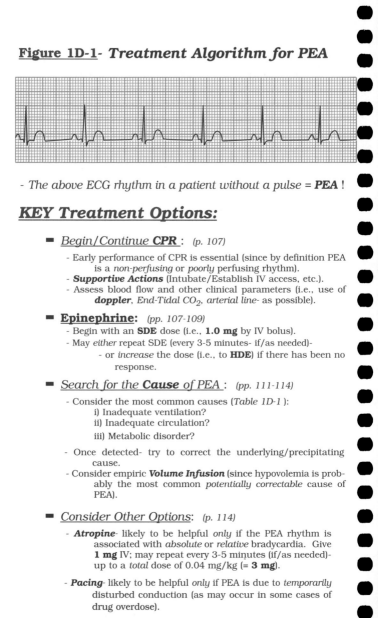

*- The above ECG rhythm in a patient without a pulse = **PEA** !*

KEY Treatment Options:

- *Begin/Continue **CPR** :* *(p. 107)*
  - Early performance of CPR is essential (since by definition PEA is a *non-perfusing* or *poorly* perfusing rhythm).
  - ***Supportive Actions*** (Intubate/Establish IV access, etc.).
  - Assess blood flow and other clinical parameters (i.e., use of ***doppler***, *End-Tidal CO_2*, *arterial line*- as possible).

- **Epinephrine:** *(pp. 107-109)*
  - Begin with an **SDE** dose (i.e., **1.0 mg** by IV bolus).
  - May *either* repeat SDE (every 3-5 minutes- if/as needed)-
    - or *increase* the dose (i.e., to **HDE**) if there has been no response.

- *Search for the **Cause** of PEA :* *(pp. 111-114)*
  - Consider the most common causes (*Table 1D-1*):
    - i) Inadequate ventilation?
    - ii) Inadequate circulation?
    - iii) Metabolic disorder?
  - Once detected- try to correct the underlying/precipitating cause.
  - Consider empiric ***Volume Infusion*** (since hypovolemia is probably the most common *potentially correctable* cause of PEA).

- *Consider Other Options:* *(p. 114)*
  - ***Atropine***- likely to be helpful *only* if the PEA rhythm is associated with *absolute* or *relative* bradycardia. Give **1 mg** IV; may repeat every 3-5 minutes (if/as needed)- up to a *total* dose of 0.04 mg/kg (= **3 mg**).

  - ***Pacing***- likely to be helpful *only* if PEA is due to *temporarily* disturbed conduction (as may occur in some cases of drug overdose).

Search for the Cause (and Potential Cure) of PEA

As already emphasized- success in the treatment of PEA most often depends on identifying and correcting the underlying (precipitating) cause of the disorder. Remember the three major categories of potential etiologies:

i) PEA rhythms due to **Inadequate Ventilation**.

ii) PEA rhythms due to **Inadequate Circulation**.

iii) PEA rhythms due to a **Metabolic Disorder**.

Specific entities in each of these categories are listed in Table 1D-1. Practically speaking, if PEA results from rupture of an aortic aneurysm or massive pulmonary embolism- there will be little one can do to save the patient. In such situations, development of PEA is most often a *preterminal* event. On the other hand, a number of *potentially reversible* causes of PEA exist that *can* be effectively treated- _IF_ they are identified in time.

Table 1D-1: *Conditions Most Likely to Cause a PEA Rhythm*

Inadequate Ventilation
- Intubation of right mainstem bronchus- or *other cause* of hypoxemia
- Tension pneumothorax (*trauma, asthma, patient on ventilator*)
- Bilateral pneumothorax (*trauma*)

Inadequate Circulation
- Pericardial effusion with tamponade (*trauma, pericarditis, uremia, too vigorous CPR*)
- Myocardial rupture or rupture of aortic aneurysm
- Massive pulmonary embolism
- **Hypovolemia** due to:
  - Acute blood loss (*trauma, GI bleeding*)
  - Dehydration
  - Septic shock
  - Cardiogenic shock (*Acute MI, myocardial contusion*)
  - Anaphylactic shock
  - Neurogenic shock (*cervical spine fracture*)

Metabolic Disorders
- Electrolyte disturbance (*severe hyperkalemia, hypokalemia, hypomagnesemia*)
- Persistent severe acidosis (*diabetic ketoacidosis, lactic acidosis*)
- Overdose of cardiac depressant drugs (*tricyclic antidepressants*)
- Hypothermia

Clinically- focus attention on specific aspects of the history and physical examination that may suggest one or more of the causes of PEA listed in Table 1D-1. Use of selected laboratory tests (either obtained from review of the patient's chart and/or ordered STAT) may provide additional clues to the underlying cause.

- *Inadequate Ventilation*. Check the patient *first* for the adequacy of respiration. Absence of breath sounds on the *left* side of the chest suggests **intubation** of the *right* **mainstem bronchus**. Simply *withdrawing* the endotracheal tube a small distance may restore bilateral breath sounds.

    If withdrawing the ET tube is not successful (and/or breath sounds are absent on the right in association with tracheal deviation)- the possibility of **tension pneumothorax** should be considered. One's index of suspicion for the presence of tension pneumothorax might be further increased in certain clinical settings (i.e., if there was a history of significant trauma, or in patients with asthma or chronic obstructive pulmonary disease- especially if they have been on a ventilator). If time does not allow for the luxury of radiographic confirmation- a *diagnostic* (and *potentially* therapeutic) tap with a large-bore needle (or Heimlich valve) may be indicated.

Note- The point of insertion for *emergency decompression* of *suspected* **tension pneumothorax** is in the second or third intercostal space. Pass the large bore (16 or 18 gauge) needle *over the top* of the rib (to avoid the intercostal vessels that run along the lower border of each rib)- and insert the needle in the *midclavicular line* (to avoid the internal mammary artery that lies medially). Air under tension produces a hissing sound- and *dramatic improvement* in the patient's hemodynamic condition should *immediately* follow.

- *Inadequate Circulation*. Direct attention to evaluating the status of the patient's circulation. Specifically, the **adequacy of intravascular volume** should be assessed. Clinically, this may be done by attempting to answer the following questions:

  - Was the patient *dehydrated* prior to the arrest?
  - Is the patient in *cardiogenic shock* (i.e., from massive acute infarction)?
  - Was the patient at risk for *pulmonary embolus*?
  - Was there a known *aortic aneurysm*?
  - Could the patient have been in *septic shock*?

> **KEY**- Practically speaking, **hypovolemia** is probably the most common (and one of the more easily treatable) causes of PEA. With this in mind, even *without* any obvious reason for hypovolemia-**empiric volume infusion** (in the form of a ≈500-1,000 ml fluid challenge) should be strongly considered at this point.

- *Cardiac Tamponade*. Acute decompensation may result if pericardial effusion develops and leads to cardiac tamponade. If the possibility of **cardiac tamponade** is at all suggested, either by history (i.e., significant chest trauma, known uremia or pericarditis)- by the course of resuscitation (i.e., suspicion of fractured ribs as a complication of too vigorous CPR)- and/or by physical examination (presence of jugular venous distention or muffled heart sounds)- then *pericardiocentesis* should be attempted. *Withdrawing as little as 50 ml of fluid under these circumstances may be lifesaving.*

> **Note**- Performance of **emergency pericardiocentesis** is best done through a subxiphoid approach- with insertion of the needle at a 20° to 30° angle with respect to the frontal plane. The needle should be directed toward the tip of the left shoulder. Aspiration is continuously applied. Entry into the pericardium usually produces a distinct "giving" sensation that should be followed by the appearance of *nonclotting* blood in the syringe. If the blood clots, it most likely has been removed from the right ventricle.

■ <u>*Metabolic disorders*</u>. Table 1D-1 lists a number of
   metabolic disorders that may also predispose to
   development of PEA. Laboratory evaluation (i.e.,
   with ABGs and STAT serum electrolytes) will
   assess some of these possibilities. The history may
   suggest others. Examples include:

   - **Persistent acidosis** (i.e., diabetic ketoacidosis, lac-
     tic acidosis)
   - Severe **electrolyte disturbance** (i.e., hyperkalemia,
     hypokalemia, or hypomagnesemia)
   - **Drug overdose** (from myocardial depressant drugs)
   - **Hypothermia** (which can be *subtle*- and ever so
     easy to overlook if the patient's temperature is
     never taken).

Other Treatment Options: *Atropine and Pacing*

Because bradycardia is *not* the principal problem with PEA-
treatment with Atropine and/or pacing will usually *not* restore
perfusion. Use of these modalities should probably be reserved
for the following situations:

i) When the rate of the PEA rhythm is *slow* (i.e., either
   absolute or relative bradycardia)- in which case both
   Atropine and **pacing** may be tried.

ii) With certain types of drug overdose, in which a healthy
    myocardium exists, but conduction is temporarily
    impaired by ingestion of one or more myocardial
    depressant drugs. In this case, implementation of
    cardiac pacing until the effect of the drug(s) wears off
    may be a lifesaving intervention.

<u>Figure 1D-2</u>- *Treatment Algorithm for Asystole*

> **<u>Is the Rhythm Truly Asystole?</u>** *(p. 117)*
> - Pulseless and unresponsive pt?
> - Monitoring leads correctly hooked up?
> - Flat line recording in *more* than 1 lead?

■ <u>Begin/Continue **CPR**</u> : *(p. 118)*

- **Supportive Actions** (Intubate/Establish IV access, etc.).

■ <u>Search for a possible **Cause(s)** of Asystole</u>

- Potential causes (and many of the treatments) of asystole are similar to those of PEA (*Table 1D-1 on p. 111*).

KEY Treatment Options:

■ <u>Consider Immediate use of **TransCutaneous Pacing (TCP)**</u> *(pp. 118-119)*
- To be effective, TCP *must* be started *early* !
- *IF available*- TCP should therefore be applied *immediately* in the treatment of asystole (either *before* or *simultaneously* with the use of drugs!).

■ **<u>Epinephrine:</u>** *(pp. 119-120)*
- Begin with an **SDE** dose (i.e., **1.0 mg** by IV bolus).
- May *either* repeat SDE (every 3-5 minutes- if/as needed)-
- or *increase* the dose (i.e., to **HDE**) if there has been no response.

■ **<u>Atropine:</u>** *(p. 120)*
- Give **1 mg** IV; May repeat every 3-5 minutes- *if/as needed* (up to a *total* dose of 0.04 mg/kg ≈**3 mg**).

■ <u>Consider Other Options</u>: *(pp. 120-121)*
- *Aminophylline*- 250 mg IV over 1-2 minutes; may repeat. (Although use of this drug is *not* yet approved by AHA Guidelines- it *might* be considered if all else fails.)
- **Sodium Bicarbonate**- indications for use in asystole are generally quite limited (i.e., to *hyperkalemia*- severe *preexisting* and/or *bicarbonate-responsive acidosis*- and *tricyclic overdose*).
- Termination of efforts . . . .

Treatment Algorithm for Asystole

AHA recommendations for treatment of **Asystole** are summarized in the algorithm we present in <u>Figure 1D-2</u>. Unfortunately, prognosis of the patient who is found in this rhythm is never good. Nevertheless, a well defined treatment protocol has been described- and on occasion, may result in successful resuscitation.

An important point to emphasize is that ultimate outcome is not necessarily as bleak when asystole occurs *in* the hospital setting- as when this rhythm is seen as the primary mechanism of cardiac arrest that occurs in the field (i.e., *outside* of the hospital). Asystole that occurs outside of the hospital setting is most often a *preterminal* rhythm that results from deterioration of V Fib in patients with prolonged cardiac arrest. Resuscitation of such patients may sometimes restore a pulse temporarily- but meaningful long-term survival (i.e., with intact neurologic function) is rare.

In contrast, asystole that develops *within* the hospital setting may reflect a somewhat different process- and may be the *direct result* of a sudden massive discharge of *parasympathetic* activity. In such cases, the rhythm may sometimes be surprisingly responsive to Atropine. This phenomenon (of sudden massive parasympathetic discharge) is most likely to be seen with certain operative procedures (i.e., endoscopy or cardiac catheterization), induction of anesthesia, toxic drug reactions, vasovagal episodes, and/or with AV block from acute *inferior* infarction.

An additional reason for the less uniformly dismal prognosis of asystole in the hospital setting is that the time elapsed from the onset of this rhythm until discovery of the patient by trained personnel tends to be much less than when asystole occurs outside of the hospital. As a result, irreversible pathophysiologic changes may not yet have set in. Such patients are therefore more likely to respond to the treatment measures described below.

> **Bottom Line**- Although long-term prognosis for patients with asystole is never good- the best chance for meaningful survival (i.e., with intact neurologic function) will be in those patients for whom the rhythm is promptly recognized- and for whom treatment is *immediately* started.

Is the Rhythm *truly* Asystole?

The diagnosis of asystole is made from the electrocardio-graphic finding of a flat line recording in *all* monitoring leads-that occurs in a patient who is *pulseless*. It is important to remember that conditions *other than* asystole may also produce a flat line recording. The differential diagnosis of a **FLAT line recording** should therefore include the following (AHA Text- Pg 1-14):

- **Fine V Fib**- that may occasionally **"masquerade"** as asystole.

- **Loose electrode leads** (or leads *not* connected to the monitor).

- **No power** (for whatever technical reason).

- **Signal gain turned down** (to a point so low that it fails to produce a rhythm on the monitor).

The reason why fine V Fib may sometimes "masquerade" as asystole relates to the fact that when the lead being monitored is *perpendicular* to the predominant vector of the fibrillation rhythm, an *isoelectric* complex (in this case, a *flat* line) will be seen. Practically speaking, this phenomenon is *not* a common occurrence.

Recognition of asystole used to be indication for delivery of an unsynchronized countershock- on the grounds that the rhythm "might possibly be V Fib" (masquerading as asystole)- and in the belief that shocking asystole "can't make the rhythm worse". *This practice is no longer justified* (AHA Text- Pg 1-23). Shocking asystole *can* make the rhythm worse- by "stunning" the heart and producing more damage to an already impaired con-duction system that may reduce even further the chance for return of spontaneous activity (AHA Text- Pg 4-7).

- Practically speaking- operator (and/or technical) errors are a much more common cause of **"false asystole"** than isoelectric V Fib masquerading as this rhythm.

- The issue of whether or not electrical activity is present can be quickly resolved- simply by *rotating* quick look paddles by 90° (or for the monitored patient, by view-ing the rhythm in *more* than a single monitoring lead).

> **Bottom Line**- Recognition of a flat line record-
> ing in a single monitoring lead does *not* justify rou-
> tine defibrillation. Instead it should prompt clinical
> reevaluation of the patient (to ensure the *true*
> absence of a pulse)- check of additional leads (to
> verify *complete* lack of electrical activity)- and
> reassessment of patient and monitor lead hook-up
> (to rule out the possibility of technical errors).

CPR/Supportive Actions/Search for a Cause

Obviously there is no perfusion with asystole. As a result-
CPR must be performed for as long as this rhythm persists.
Other **Supportive Actions** (i.e., intubation, establishment of IV
access, etc.) should be accomplished at the earliest opportunity.

As was the case for PEA- always consider the possibility of
an *underlying* cause that might predispose to development of this
rhythm. Potential causes of asystole are similar to those that are
likely to precipitate PEA (*See Table 1D-1*). When such factors are
responsible for the rhythm- success in treatment will depend on
identifying and correcting this underlying cause.

> **Note**- Patients with bradyasystolic arrest that
> occurs in association with **special circumstances**
> (i.e., *hypothermia- electrocution- drug overdose-
> drowning- sudden failure of a permanent pacemaker*)
> represent a special group, for whom prognosis may
> even be favorable- *IF* the patient is promptly attend-
> ed to. This is because underlying the rhythm dis-
> order, the myocardium of such individuals may be
> relatively normal. As a result- *greater persistence in
> resuscitative efforts is usually appropriate* (in the
> hope of providing *supportive care* while precipitat-
> ing factors are identified and treated).

Use of Pacing for Asystole

In general, pacemaker therapy is only effective in the treatment of bradycardia and asystole when myocardial function has
been at least to some extent preserved. As a result, it is unlikely

to be helpful in the treatment of asystole when this rhythm occurs as a preterminal event after prolonged (and unsuccessful) attempts at resuscitation. In acknowledgement of the almost uniformly dismal prognosis of such patients- AHA Guidelines emphasize that pacing is now an *optional* procedure that need *not* always be tried in such situations (AHA Text- Pg 1-23).

- Pacemaker therapy is most likely to be successful in the treatment of bradyasystolic cardiac arrest if attempted *early* in the process (i.e., *before* irreversibility has set in). As a result, if it is to be used- **TCP** (**T**rans-**C**utaneous **P**acing) should be applied as soon as the device is available- which may be *before* (and/or *simultaneously* with) the use of drugs (AHA Text- Pg 1-24).

- Pacemaker therapy is *no longer recommended* as routine treatment for patients with bradyasystolic cardiac arrest. Special attention should be given to the decision of whether to even attempt pacing in patients with out-of-hospital cardiac arrest who have not responded to other measures- especially when the period of arrest has been prolonged. The sombering reality is that long-term prognosis for most of these patients is dismal- *regardless* of what interventions are undertaken. AHA Guidelines suggest that pacing actually becomes **relatively *contraindicated* when delay** before initiation of treatment with this modality **exceeds 20 minutes**- since the chance for successful resuscitation with intact neurologic function is virtually nil in this situation (AHA Text- Pg 5-2).

Use of Epinephrine

The initial drug of choice for the treatment of asystole is **Epinephrine**. Because the vasoconstrictor effect of Epinephrine in the arrested heart makes it the *KEY* pharmacologic agent for favoring blood flow to the coronary and cerebral circulation- the drug should be used *liberally* in the treatment of asystole.

- AHA Guidelines recommend *beginning* with an **SDE** dose of Epinephrine (i.e., **1 mg IV**). This dose may be repeated every 3-5 minutes for as long as the patient remains in asystole.

- Consideration should be given to increasing the dose of Epinephrine if the patient fails to respond to one or more doses of SDE. Practically speaking- you *can't* really overdose on Epinephrine when treating asystole (i.e., *"You can't be deader than dead"*). Escalation of the dose (i.e., to **HDE**) is therefore appropriate- for *potentially salvageable* patients who are felt to have a reasonable chance for restoration of intact neurologic function. AHA Guidelines leave the decision of whether or not to escalate the dose of Epinephrine entirely at the discretion of the treating clinician (AHA Text- Pg 7-4).

Use of Atropine

As noted above- asystole may occasionally be caused by a sudden massive discharge of *parasympathetic* activity. As a result, treatment with *Atropine* should always be tried.

- The *initial* recommended dose of Atropine for treatment of asystole is **1.0 mg IV**. This dose may be repeated every 3-5 minutes if there is no response (up to a *total* dose of 0.04 mg/kg- or ≈**3 mg** for an *average-sized* adult).

- AHA Guidelines allow for use of Atropine at even more frequent intervals than every 3-5 minutes in the treatment of bradyasystolic cardiac arrest. Thus, the drug can be given at *1-minute* intervals in this situation (AHA Text- Pg 1-30).

- Practically speaking- the chance that Atropine will work in asystole is relatively small. This is particularly true when the drug is used in the treatment of prolonged out-of-hospital cardiac arrest.

When All Else Fails: *Use of Aminophylline?*

Although *not* included in AHA Guidelines, a drug to consider when all else fails (i.e., for what would *otherwise* be *lethal* bradyasystolic arrest) is **Aminophylline**. Data on use of this agent for treatment of asystole are limited- but promising. The theory proposed to account for the beneficial effect of

Aminophylline in this situation relates to potential mediation of severe ischemia and bradycardia/asystole by release of *endogenous adenosine* (in the body's attempt to vasodilate and restore myocardial oxygen supply). As a result, endogenous adenosine may accumulate- leading to further exacerbation of ischemia (by a "coronary steal" phenomenon) and/or contributing to (or causing) more profound bradycardia/asystole. The mechanism by which Aminophylline works may therefore result from the known *antagonistic* effect that this drug exerts on adenosine.

- If you decide to use Aminophylline- the dose we suggest is **250 mg IV**, to be given over 1-2 minutes. This dose may be repeated if there is no response.

> **Bottom Line**- Clearly, additional studies are needed. Nevertheless, it is difficult to imagine how administration of Aminophylline could worsen the prognosis of refractory asystolic cardiac arrest. *Consideration might therefore be given to empiric use of this drug for this otherwise almost certainly lethal condition.*

Use of Sodium Bicarbonate for Asystole

Indications for use of **Sodium Bicarbonate** in the treatment of asystole are limited. They include *hyperkalemia*- severe *pre-existing* and/or *bicarbonate-responsive acidosis* (that is thought to have contributed to or precipitated the arrest)- and *tricyclic overdose*. Empiric use of Sodium Bicarbonate is no longer recommended in cardiac arrest.

Consider Termination of Efforts

AHA Guidelines intentionally *avoid* citing a time limit beyond which resuscitation will never be successful. Instead, they emphasize how "*special situations call for common sense and clinical judgement* " (AHA Text- Pg 1-25). Practically speaking, the prognosis of patients with out-of-hospital bradyasystolic arrest is exceedingly poor- especially if the patient fails to respond to initial attempts at resuscitation. In such situations- "asystole most often represents a *confirmation of death*- rather than a rhythm to be treated". *Resuscitation efforts may therefore be stopped*- after intubation, IV access, basic CPR, and a trial of Atropine/Epinephrine. A trial of pacing is *not* necessarily indicated for all patients.

Figure 1D-3- *Treatment Algorithm for Bradycardia*

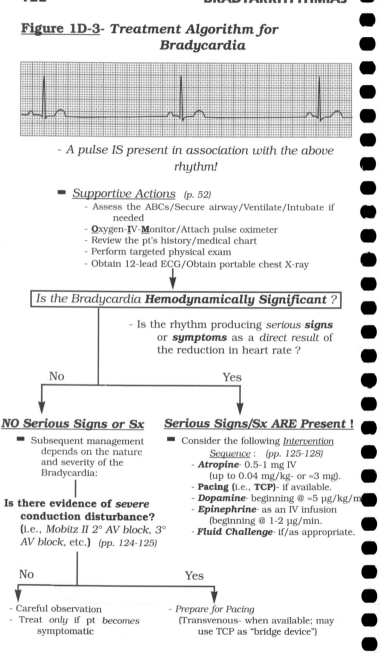

- A pulse IS present in association with the above rhythm!

- **■ *Supportive Actions*** *(p. 52)*
  - Assess the ABCs/Secure airway/Ventilate/Intubate if needed
  - **O**xygen-**I**V-**M**onitor/Attach pulse oximeter
  - Review the pt's history/medical chart
  - Perform targeted physical exam
  - Obtain 12-lead ECG/Obtain portable chest X-ray

---

*Is the Bradycardia **Hemodynamically Significant** ?*

*- Is the rhythm producing serious **signs** or **symptoms** as a direct result of the reduction in heart rate ?*

No   Yes

NO Serious Signs or Sx

- ■ Subsequent management depends on the nature and severity of the Bradycardia:

Is there evidence of *severe* conduction disturbance?
(i.e., *Mobitz II 2° AV block, 3° AV block,* etc.) *(pp. 124-125)*

No   Yes

- Careful observation
- Treat *only* if pt *becomes* symptomatic

Serious Signs/Sx ARE Present !

- ■ Consider the following <u>*Intervention Sequence*</u> : *(pp. 125-128)*
  - ***Atropine***- 0.5-1 mg IV
    (up to 0.04 mg/kg- or ≈3 mg).
  - **Pacing (i.e., TCP)**- if available.
  - ***Dopamine***- beginning @ ≈5 µg/kg/m
  - ***Epinephrine***- as an IV infusion (beginning @ 1-2 µg/min.
  - ***Fluid Challenge***- if/as appropriate.

- *Prepare for Pacing*
  (Transvenous- when available; may use TCP as "bridge device")

Treatment Algorithm for Bradycardia

AHA recommendations for treatment of **Bradycardia** are summarized in the algorithm we present in Figure 1D-3. For the purpose of this algorithm- the term **Bradycardia** is used to encompass the diverse group of cardiac rhythms that are unified by the finding of a *slow* ventricular rate (i.e., of *less* than **60 beats/minute**). The principal entities included within this group are the following:

- *Sinus bradycardia* (which often occurs in conjunction with *sinus arrhythmia*).
- *A Fib* with a *slow* ventricular response.
- The various forms of AV block.
- *Escape rhythms* (including *junctional* escape and *slow* idioventricular rhythm).
- Rhythms that manifest **"relative" bradycardia** (for which the heart rate is *inappropriately slow* for the clinical situation at hand- *despite* the fact that the rate may be somewhat faster than 60 beats/minute).

Is the Rhythm Hemodynamically Significant?

Once told that a pulse is present (as we are at the top of Figure 1D-3)- **Supportive Actions** should be accomplished (as feasible, given the clinical situation). While this is being done, attention is directed at answering the *KEY* Clinical Question: **Is the rhythm hemodynamically significant**? Specifically, one seeks to determine if the bradyarrhythmia is causing the patient problems as a *direct result* of the reduction in heart rate. There are two possibilities:

i) **NO Serious Signs or Symptoms result from the Bradycardia.** In this case, subsequent management will depend on the nature and severity of the bradycardia. In general- no immediate intervention (other than careful observation) should be needed (since the patient is *not* symptomatic). Preparation may need to be made for pacing (and/or for pacing *back-up*- known as **"anticipatory pacing readiness"**)- depending on whether or not there is evidence of *severe* conduction disturbance. The advantage of using **TCP** (**T**rans**C**utaneous **P**acing) in this situation is that the device may be placed on the patient in *standby* mode (i.e., applied to the patient- but with pacing *not* turned on).

ii) _Serious Signs or Symptoms ARE present._ In this case, immediate intervention *is* needed (since the patient *is* symptomatic!). AHA Guidelines suggest the intervention sequence that we show in Figure 1D-3.

KEY- Always **treat the patient- NOT the monitor!** (AHA Text- Pg 1-30). Much more important than whether a slow rhythm is the result of 2° or 3° AV block- or simply profound sinus bradycardia (as seen in Figure 1C-3)- will be the patient's clinical condition and hemodynamic status (i.e., effective heart rate, blood pressure, mental status, presence or absence of symptoms). Treatment of bradycardia (with drugs and/or pacing) may sometimes need to be started when the patient is symptomatic *without* being sure of what the specific diagnosis of the rhythm is. In reality, diagnosis of the rhythm should proceed *simultaneously* with initiation of therapy (AHA Text- Pg 1-30)- with realization that from a practical standpoint, a patient with serious signs or symptoms from severe bradycardia will *initially* be treated the same (i.e., with Atropine, pacing, Dopamine, and/or Epinephrine)- *regardless* of what the specific type of bradycardia happens to be.

From a clinical perspective- determination of the specific ECG diagnosis of the type of bradycardia becomes more important in the decision making process when the patient is hemodynamically stable. In this situation, determination of the need for pacemaker therapy will depend on the severity of the conduction disturbance. In general, pacing will be needed for patients with **Mobitz II 2° AV block** and/or **3° AV block with QRS widening**. Insight to the expected clinical course and response to therapy for patients with acute infarction and new-onset conduction system disorders may be provided by consideration of the site of infarction (AHA Text- Pg 1-32):

- Patients with acute **_anterior_ infarction** who develop new-onset 2° AV block (which is typically of the Mobitz II type) or 3° AV block (which will typically manifest a *wide* QRS complex escape rhythm)- generally require transvenous pacing. This is because these conduction system disorders are usually *not* reversible. Atropine should *only* be used in such patients with extreme caution (if it is used at all). TCP may prove invaluable as a *"bridge"* device until transvenous pacing is available.

■ In contrast, patients with acute ***inferior* infarction** typically manifest a *narrow* QRS complex escape rhythm- since the anatomic level of AV block is most often at the level of the AV node with this type of infarction. As a result, these patients generally respond well to Atropine (which opposes the vagotonic activity that most often causes the conduction defect). Fortunately, 2° AV block (most often Mobitz I) and 3° AV block that occur in association with acute *inferior* infarction are usually *transient* conduction disorders that are likely to *spontaneously* resolve in time). If symptoms are minimal or absent- *standby* use of TCP may be all that is needed in the interim.

Symptomatic Bradycardia: *Rationale for Intervention Sequence*

Many factors enter into the decision making process for the treatment of bradycardia. In the hope of optimizing the ***Intervention Sequence*-** we emphasize the following points:

■ The need for specific interventions in the treatment of bradycardia should be based on the *severity* of the clinical situation (AHA Text- Pg 1-30). AHA Guidelines emphasize that rather than slow and discrete stepwise progression through a well defined protocol- rapid decision making and **near simultaneous implementation of *multiple* interventions may be needed** (AHA Text- Pg 1-31). For example, the patient with severe symptomatic bradycardia may receive Atropine *at the same time* as preparation is made for cardiac pacing. Preparation may also be made at this time for IV infusion of Dopamine (and/or Epinephrine) in anticipation of the possibility that Atropine may be ineffective and application of TCP could be delayed.

- *If Signs/Symptoms from Bradycardia are "Mild"*- AHA Guidelines suggest selection of **Atropine** as the initial pharmacologic intervention "of choice" (AHA Text-Pg 1-30). The dose recommended in this situation is **0.5-1 mg IV**- which may be repeated every 3-5 minutes as needed (up to a *total* dose of 0.04 mg/kg- or ≈**3 mg**).

    - The lower dose of Atropine (i..e, **0.5 mg**) is preferable for *initial* treatment of the patient with less severe symptoms from the bradycardia. Consider increasing the dose (i.e., to **1.0 mg**) if the patient fails to respond to one or two 0.5 mg doses- and/or if the symptoms from bradycardia become more severe.

> **Note**- Use of Atropine is *not* benign. By blocking parasympathetic output, the drug may *unmask* previously contained enhanced sympathetic activity. This may lead to development of *tachycardia* and/or precipitation of potentially malignant ventricular arrhythmias (including VT and V Fib).
>
> **Bottom Line**- Atropine should *not* be used to treat the asymptomatic patient with bradycardia. Instead, use of the drug should be reserved for treatment of *symptomatic* bradycardia (i.e., bradycardia associated with chest pain or dyspnea)- and/or bradycardia accompanied by signs of *hemodynamic compromise* (i.e., hypotension, heart failure, ventricular ectopy, or altered mental status).

    - Although one usually waits at least 3-5 minutes before repeating the dose of Atropine- the drug may be dosed more frequently (i.e., as often as every 1-3 minutes!) for selected patients with *marked* hemodynamic compromise from the slow rate (AHA Text- Pg 1-30).

    - Atropine should be used with extreme caution (if at all) when the rhythm being treated is advanced AV block with ventricular escape (i.e., with a wide QRS complex). Theoretically, Atropine could even *worsen* hemodynamic status in such patients (if by increasing the atrial rate it reduced the number of impulses conducted to the ventricles). Pacing appears to be preferable for such patients- especially if the AV block occurs in association with acute *anterior* infarction (AHA Text- Pg 1-32).

- The denervated (transplanted) heart will *not* respond to Atropine. As a result, one should immediately intervene with either pacing and/or catecholamine infusion in such patients.

- *If Symptoms are "More Severe"*- Consideration should be given to ***pacing*** as soon as this modality is available. AHA Guidelines emphasize that it *IS* appropriate to use ***TCP*** as the *initial* intervention in the treatment sequence- *IF* the bradycardia is severe and/or the clinical condition is unstable (AHA Text- Pg 1-31). Pacing is also *preferable* to Atropine when the rhythm being treated is advanced AV block with ventricular escape (for the reasons stated above).

  - Pacing should *not* be delayed while attempting to achieve IV access (or while waiting for Atropine to take effect)- *especially if the patient is symptomatic* (AHA Text- Pg 1-29).

  - Although admittedly, pacing is *not* very effective in the treatment of bradyasystolic cardiac arrest- it is generally much more effective (and may be *lifesaving*) when used to treat patients who *have* a pulse and who manifest symptomatic bradycardia. Because the primary problem in such patients is the slow rate- cardiac pacing would seem to be the *ideal* modality for responding to this situation.

  - Keep in mind that it will *not* always be possible to implement external pacing (i.e., awake patients may not always tolerate the device; electrical capture with effective mechanical contraction may not always be obtained).

■ *If Atropine is Ineffective and Pacing is Unavailable-* Consider the use of a pressor agent. With *less* severe symptoms- ***Dopamine*** is the agent that is generally preferred in this situation. AHA Guidelines suggest beginning at a dose of **5 µg/kg/minute**- and titrating the rate of infusion upward as needed according to the clinical response (AHA Text- Pg 1-31).

If hemodynamic symptoms are more severe- AHA Guidelines suggest beginning directly with **IV infusion** of ***Epinephrine*** (instead of Dopamine). The initial rate recommended for IV infusion of Epinephrine is **1-2 µg/minute**- which can be rapidly titrated upward as needed according to the clinical response.

> **Note**- Epinephrine should *not* be given by IV bolus when using the drug as a *pressor* agent (i.e., to treat a patient who is *not* in cardiac arrest). Use of continuous IV infusion provides the advantage of *moment-to-moment* titration capability for altering the dose of drug given. Should an adverse effect occur, the IV infusion can *immediately* be turned down (or off). In contrast, if Epinpehrine is given by IV bolus and an adverse effect occurs- *"You can't take the bolus back."*

Additional Considerations/Pitfalls

In addition to standard recommendations for treatment of bradycardia that are listed above, a number of thoughts should be kept in mind:

i) Bradycardia will *not* always be the result of conduction system disease. Correction of other factors (i.e., *hypoxemia- hypovolemia- electrolyte disturbance-* etc.) may sometimes be all that is needed to "cure" the problem. This point emphasizes the importance of always considering the "**D**" component (i.e., ***D****ifferential* ***D****iagnosis*) of the **Secondary Survey**- especially when confronted with an arrhythmia that does not respond to standard treatment measures.

ii) Patients with bradycardia and hypotension may be ***volume depleted***- either from volume loss (due to hemorrhage or dehydration), or as a result of inappropriate vasodilatation (from acute myocardial infarction, septic or neurogenic shock).

- Although most of the time, patients with hypotension will be *tachycardic*- this is *not* always the case. In particular, patients with acute *inferior* infarction frequently manifest excessive parasympathetic tone- which commonly leads to bradycardia and hypotension.

- Clinically, it will often be difficult to adequately assess volume status. As a result, it is important to always maintain a high index of suspicion for the possibility of hypovolemia. Placing such patients in Trendelenburg position, and cautious administration of a ***fluid challenge*** (with **150-500 ml** of normal saline) is the treatment of choice.

Note- An extremely common problem in emergency cardiac care is **hypotension**. It is important to realize that patients with hypotension may be tachycardic, bradycardic- or have a normal heart rate. Optimal management ideally entails identification and correction of the underlying cause of the hypotension. Although this goal often extends beyond immediate capabilities of the emergency care provider (who is faced with the problem of keeping alive a patient in extremis)- the point to emphasize is that ***empiric* volume infusion** should *always* be strongly considered as a *potential* therapeutic intervention for patients with hypotension of uncertain etiology- especially if they fail to respond to standard treatment measures.

---

iii) As we suggest in our section on asystole (on page 120)- administration of **Aminophylline** might also be *considered* as a treatment alternative for the patient with *severe* bradycardia who fails to respond to more standard measures (i.e., *Atropine*, *Epinephrine*, and *TCP*).

- If you decide to use Aminophylline- the dose we suggest is **250 mg IV**, to be given over a 1-2 minute period. This dose may be repeated if there is no response.

> **Note**- Use of Aminophylline is *not* yet included in AHA Guidelines. Standard measures should clearly be tried first. Nevertheless- if the patient remains symptomatic from severe bradycardia *despite* standard measures- consideration *might* be given to the use of this drug.

iv) Do *not* use **Lidocaine** as a prophylactic measure (to prevent V Fib) if the patient is in advanced AV block with ventricular escape beats (and/or a ventricular escape rhythm). In this situation- Lidocaine may abolish the *only* escape rhythm you have!

v) Use of **Isoproterenol** as a pressor agent has been strongly discouraged in recent years. This is because of the drug's potential to produce deleterious effects on the heart and circulation (including peripheral vasodilatation and an *increase* in myocardial oxygen consumption). If used at all (as it occasionally may be to provide *pure* chronotropic support)- the dose of Isoproterenol must be kept *low*- and extreme *caution* is urged! We emphasize that at the present time- *other* pressor agents (i.e., Dopamine, Epinephrine) *are clearly preferred* to the use of Isoproterenol (AHA Text- Pg 1-32).

vi) Clinical judgement is needed to determine whether **CPR** should be performed on the patient with bradycardia *in addition* to other therapeutic measures. The need to perform CPR clearly depends on the *severity* of hypotension and the degree of hemodynamic compromise. It is obviously *not* needed for treatment of mild bradycardia- or even for 2° or 3° AV block if the patient is alert and asymptomatic. On the other hand, continuation of CPR would be an essential component of therapy for an unresponsive patient in a slow ventricular escape rhythm with marked hypotension. *Whether to perform CPR in less clearcut situations is a matter of clinical judgement.*

Questions to Further Understanding

Why Should Use of Atropine be Reserved for Treatment of Patients with Evidence of Hemodynamic Compromise?

Treatment with Atropine is *not* benign. As a result, it is generally best to withhold use of this drug *unless* the patient is clearly symptomatic. Adverse effects that may be associated (at least on occasion) with use of this parasympatholytic agent include:

- an *"unmasking"* of previously opposed (and underlying) *sympathetic hyperactivity* that could result in excessive tachycardia and/or precipitate ventricular arrhythmias (including VT/V Fib).

- *acceleration of the supraventricular response*- which could paradoxically exacerbate the degree of AV block (since the AV node may not be able to conduct as many impulses at the faster rate).

Is Use of a Pacemaker Preferable to Atropine for Treatment of Hemodynamically Significant Bradyarrhythmias?

Cardiac pacing is the treatment of choice for hemodynamically significant bradyarrhythmias that occur in the setting of cardiac arrest. The problem with *transvenous* pacing is that the insertion procedure is invasive, takes time, and requires the presence of a skilled operator. Advantages of **T**rans**C**utaneous **P**acing (***TCP***) is that it is easy to apply, takes only seconds, and is completely noninvasive.

As emphasized previously, treatment with Atropine is *not* benign. As a result, use of TCP may be preferred to Atropine therapy if the device is immediately available- especially if the bradycardia is severe and/or the clinical condition is unstable (AHA Text- Pg 1-31).

> **Note**- Practically speaking, a transcutaneous
> pacemaker may not always be immediately avail-
> able when the need arises. Because of the rapidity
> with which a dose of Atropine may be administered-
> it *is* reasonable to try this treatment first (if the
> patient is symptomatic) while sending for the pace-
> maker.
>
> **Bottom Line**- Near *simultaneous* implementa-
> tion of *multiple* interventions is appropriate in an
> arrest situation (AHA Text- Pg 1-31). Clinical judge-
> ment is needed (and encouraged!) to determine the
> most appropriate intervention(s) for a given situation.

Why is it Preferable to Administer Epinephrine by IV Infusion for Treatment of Hemodynamically Significant Bradyarrhythmias?

The drawback of bolus administration is that once a dose of
drug has been given- *it cannot be "taken back"*. Hemodynamic
effects persist until the action of the drug wears off. In contrast,
use of a continuous IV infusion allows *moment-to-moment* titration of the dose of drug according to its clinical effect.

With respect to Epinephrine- the potent chronotropic and
inotropic effects of the drug are potentially quite arrhythmogenic
when administered to a patient with a spontaneous circulation.
Use of a continuous IV infusion allows much more careful dose
titration- as well as the ability to immediately *turn off* the infusion in the event of an adverse hemodynamic effect.

Is it Even Worth Treating Asystole?

Admittedly, the prognosis for asystole is *never* good.
Nevertheless, the outlook for this rhythm when it develops during cardiac arrest that occurs *in* the hospital- is *not* necessarily
as bleak as when asystole is the primary mechanism of a cardiac
arrest occurring *outside* of the hospital. Asystole in this latter
setting is most often a *preterminal* rhythm that arises after V Fib
deteriorates. In contrast, asystole occurring in a hospital setting

may occasionally result from massive parasympathetic dis-
charge- and consequently, may be surprisingly responsive to
Atropine therapy. In addition, time until discovery is usually
much less for in-hospital asystole- so that the rhythm may occasionally respond to Epinephrine or early institution of pacing.

What is the Maximal Dose of Epinephrine for Treatment of Asystole?

There is no maximal dose of Epinephrine for this indication.
Epinephrine is the *one* drug (and perhaps the *only* drug) that will
favor perfusion to the heart and brain in the setting of cardiac
arrest. Practically speaking, there should be *nothing to lose* from
use of HDE in this situation- and there *may* be some patients
who respond only to higher doses of the drug. We therefore favor
consideration of *higher* doses of Epinephrine at a relatively *early*
point in the course of managing asystole- *IF* the patient is felt to
be potentially salvageable, and the rhythm has not responded to
Atropine and SDE doses of drug.

What is Meant by the Term "Anticipatory Pacing Readiness"? When Might this be More Appropriate than Actual Initiation of Pacing?

The major indication for pacing with bradycardia occurs
when the patient is felt to be symptomatic as a *direct result* of the
reduction in heart rate. However, even when heart rate is significantly slowed pacing may *not* necessarily be needed- *IF* the
patient is otherwise unaffected (i.e., normotensive and asymptomatic). Despite this, it would still seem prudent to *anticipate* the
possibility that the bradycardia might suddenly *become* hemodynamically significant (perhaps *without* warning)- especially when
the clinical setting is that of a cardiopulmonary emergency. AHA
Guidelines therefore allow that "in conscious patients with *hemodynamically stable* bradycardia it may be *reasonable* to attach
electrodes to the patient - and leave the pacemaker in **Standby
Mode** "- ready to turn on at *any* moment- *IF* the patient's condition were to deteriorate at *any* time during the treatment process
(AHA Text- Pg 5-3).

- The advantages of **anticipatory pacing readiness** (i.e., use of TCP in the *Standby Mode*)- are that it may obviate the need for transvenous pacing (which is an invasive procedure)- and/or *minimize* the time needed to implement TCP if hemodynamic decompensation suddenly occurs.

- *Pacing readiness* is especially appropriate for patients with bradyarrhythmias that are likely to either resolve on their own or with treatment (i.e., *drug-induced* bradycardia).   It is also appropriate for treatment of *new* 2° or 3° AV block- and/or *new* bifascicular block- that occurs in the setting of Acute MI in a *hemodynamically stable* patient (AHA Text- Pg 5-2).

Note- If the decision is made to use TCP in the *Standby Mode*- it may be advisable to verify that mechanical capture is possible, and that the patient will be able to *tolerate* pacing in the event it is needed (AHA Text- Pg 1-32 and Pg 5-5).

ADDENDUM

Pediatric Resuscitation

Pediatric resuscitation is a topic unto itself. Although full discussion of this issue is best reserved for comprehensive review in an AHA/AAP (American Academy of Pediatrics) course in *Pediatric Advanced Life Support* (i.e., **PALS**)- we include a brief section in this book on the most important drugs used in pediatric resuscitation because: 1) Adult ACLS providers are likely to at least *occasionally* encounter cardiopulmonary emergencies in children; and 2) Dosing considerations for the drugs used in pediatric resuscitation are very different than for use of the same drugs in adults. Ready reference to a source of information on drugs used in pediatric resuscitation may greatly facilitate dose determination at the time of emergency.

Note- Dosing recommendations cited here are based on weight of the child in kilograms (kg)- with specific values provided for a **10 kg**- **20 kg**- and **30 kg** patient- and inclusion of the recommended adult dose for comparison.

Reference is periodically made in this section to the American Heart Association (AHA) Textbook in *Pediatric Advanced Life Support* (**PALS**)- Chameides L, Hazinski MF (Eds), American Heart Association, Dallas, 1994.

Overview of *KEY* Concepts in Pediatric Resuscitation

Inadequate oxygenation is the *most* common cause of cardiac arrest in children! As a result, the most important *initial focus* of cardiopulmonary resuscitation in pediatric patients *must* be to optimize ventilation/oxygenation- *rather than* administering drugs.

- The pediatric heart most often responds to hypoxemia by *slowing* the heart rate. This is why **asystole** and **bradyarrhythmias** (i.e., *sinus bradycardia- sinus node arrest* with a slow *escape* rhythm- severe bradycardia from *advanced AV block*)- are the most common **preterminal rhythms** to be seen in association with cardiopulmonary arrest in children.

■ Establishing a patent airway that allows adequate ventilation and oxygenation (*enhanced* by supplemental oxygen) is the *KEY* to success- *and will often be all that is needed.* Practically speaking then- **Oxygen** is the *most important drug* in pediatric resuscitation.

■ In addition to hypoxemia, other factors that are likely to contribute to causing pediatric cardiopulmonary arrest/arrhythmogenesis include *acidosis- hypotension- electrolyte* disturbance- *hypoglycemia- hypothermia-* and/or the presence of an *underlying illness* (i.e., sepsis, pneumonia, dehydration, etc.). Correction of **underlying disorders** is therefore the second important *KEY* for successful resuscitation in children.

■ If pharmacologic therapy *is* needed for treatment of pediatric bradycardia/asystole- **Epinephrine** is the drug of choice (*See below*). Atropine is a *second-line* agent that should probably be used *only* when symptoms are *severe* and the patient has *not* responded to other measures (*including* adequate oxygenation and Epinephrine).

Arrhythmia Interpretation: *KEY* Concepts

The intricacies of arrhythmia interpretation are far less important in the treatment of pediatric resuscitation than they are in the treatment of adults. This is because specific treatment of the rhythm per se is far less likely to be needed.

■ Practically speaking- most arrhythmias seen during pediatric resuscitation are *SUPRAventricular.* By far, the most common *mechanism* is **sinus**- and the most common rhythms seen are sinus *bradycardia- tachycardia-* or *normal* sinus rhythm.

- Differentiation between the sinus mechanism rhythms depends *both* on the patient's age as well as on the clinical condition. For example- a heart rate of 120 beats/minute should be considered as normal for children up to 2 years of age. Mean heart rate in children does not drop below 100 beats/minute until about 8 years of age. On the other hand, a seemingly "normal" heart rate of 80 beats/minute most probably reflects a **relative bradycardia** when it occurs in the setting of a cardiopulmonary arrest in a child.

- Unlike the situation in adults- **Pulseless VT/V Fib** are extremely *uncommon* arrhythmias in pediatric arrests. As a result- *defibrillation is only rarely needed in pediatric resuscitation.* (In cases when V Fib *does* occur in a child- it is almost always associated with congenital heart disease- and/or following a *prolonged* period of hypoxemia from a preceding respiratory arrest.)

- *In infants-* the most common tachyarrhythmia to produce hemodynamic instability is **PSVT** (**P**aroxysmal **S**upra**V**entricular **T**achycardia). Heart rates of infants with this rhythm may be as fast as 250-300 beats/minute. However, because sinus tachycardia may also attain heart rates of over 200 beats/minute in this age group- differentiation between sinus tachycardia and PSVT will *not* always be easy.

Epinephrine

Next to Oxygen- **Epinephrine** is the most important drug used in pediatric resuscitation. Unfortunately, the optimal dose of Epinephrine for use in pediatric resuscitation remains uncertain. Two principal factors account for this uncertainty: 1) the limited number of clinical trials that have been performed on the use of this drug in the treatment of pediatric cardiopulmonary arrest; and 2) the clinical reality that *regardless* of whatever interventions are tried- the likelihood of achieving meaningful *long-term survival* (i.e., with intact neurologic function) is exceedingly small.

Recommendations for **_Dosing of Epinephrine_** for pediatric resuscitation are based on the following premises:

- _Lower doses_ of Epinephrine (i.e., **0.01 mg/kg**) may be effective in the treatment of symptomatic bradycardia- _and should be tried first._

- Significantly _higher doses_ of Epinephrine are likely to be needed for more severe bradycardia- especially for treatment of children with asystolic or pulseless cardiac arrest. As a result, a higher dose of IV Epinephrine (i.e., **0.1 mg/kg**) should be tried after 3-5 minutes- _IF_ the patient fails to respond to the lower (i.e., 0.01 mg/kg) dose.

- Epinephrine (in appropriate doses) should be repeated on a _regular_ basis (i.e., _every_ **3-5 minutes**- as needed)- _throughout_ the resuscitative effort if the patient fails to respond to other measures.

- _If IV access cannot be achieved_- Epinephrine (as well as _Lidocaine_ and _Atropine_)- can be given by the **_E_ndo_T_racheal _(ET) route_**. Because absorption following ET administration is _less_ reliable- _higher doses_ of drug should be used than for IV administration (_See below_).

- Epinephrine (as well as _other drugs, fluids,_ and _blood_) may also be given by the **_I_ntra_O_sseous _(IO) route_**. Because absorption of drugs and fluids is _excellent_ by this route (with onset of action and peak serum levels being _comparable_ to that achieved following IV administration)- recommendations for dosing (_of both drug boluses and continuous infusions_) by the **IO route** are virtually the _same_ as recommendations for **IV dosing**.

Note- Absorption of Epinephrine following _either_ **IV** _or_ **IO** administration is superior to absorption of drug following administration by the **ET** route. As a result, _both_ IV and IO access are preferred over the ET route for drug administration. In general, if reliable IV access cannot be achieved in a child _less_ than 6 years of age _within_ 3 attempts (and/or _within_ ≈90 seconds)- _then an attempt should be made to establish_ **IO** _access_ (AHA Text- Pg 1-64).

Epinephrine Dosing- Treatment of Symptomatic Bradycardia:

- **Dose** *for **IV** or **IO*** *administration* = **0.01 mg/kg** (0.1 mL/kg of 1:10,000 solution). This dose may be repeated every 3-5 minutes (AHA PALS Text- Pg 6-6).

- **Dose** *for **ET*** *administration* = **0.1 mg/kg** (0.1 mL/kg of 1:1,000 solution). This dose may be repeated every 3-5 minutes (AHA PALS Text- Pg 6-6).

> **Note**- The dose of **Epinephrine** recommended for **ET** administration is now **10 times greater** than the dose recommended for either IV or IO adminis-tration (0.1 mg/kg *compared to* 0.01 mg/kg). However, because the *concentration* of the Epinephrine solution recommended for ET adminis-tration *also* differs by a factor of 10 (i.e., 1:1,000 soln. *instead* of 1:10,000)- the *total* amount of fluid delivered to a child of any given body weight should be the same- *regardless* of whether the drug is given by the IV, IO, or ET routes (*See Table below*).

Epinephrine Dosing: *For Treatment of Symptomatic Bradycardia*		
Weight of Patient	**Dose for IV or IO Bolus Administration** (= 0.01 mg/kg) (= 0.1 mL/kg of 1:**10,000** soln.)	**Dose for ET Administration** (= 0.1 mg/kg) (= 0.1 mL/kg of 1:**1,000** soln.)
10 kg	**0.1 mg** (1 ml of 1:10,000 soln.)	**1 mg ET** (1 ml of 1:1,000 soln.)
20 kg	**0.2 mg** (2 ml of 1:10,000 soln.)	**2 mg ET** (2 ml of 1:1,000 soln.)
30 kg	**0.3 mg** (3 ml of 1:10,000 soln.)	**3 mg ET** (3 ml of 1:1,000 soln.)
Adult Dose	**1.0 mg IV** (= SDE)	≈ **2-2.5 mg ET** (*as initial dose*)

> **Note**- New AHA recommendations that we cite on these pages advise use of *differing concentrations* of Epinephrine (i.e., use of a **1:10,000 soln.** and **1:1,000 soln.**- when giving *lower* and *higher* doses of drug, respectively). As a result- *extreme care must be taken to avoid errors in dosing* !!!

Epinephrine Dosing- Treatment of Asystole/Pulseless Arrest:

- **Initial Dose** for **IV** or **IO** administration = **0.01 mg/kg** (0.1 mL/kg of 1:10,000 solution)- *which is the SAME dose recommended for use of IV (or IO) Epinephrine in treating symptomatic Bradycardia!*

- **Initial Dose** for **ET** administration = **0.1 mg/kg** (0.1 mL/kg of 1:1,000 solution)- *which is the SAME dose recommended for use of ET Epinephrine in treating symptomatic Bradycardia!*

- **2nd (and subsequent) Doses** for **IV**, **IO**, or **ET** administration = **0.1 mg/kg** (0.1 mL/kg of 1:1,000 solution)- *given every* **3-5 minutes** *as needed.*

Epinephrine Dosing: *For Treatment of Asystolic or Pulseless Arrest*		
Weight of Patient	**Initial Dose for IV or IO Bolus Administration*** (= 0.01 mg/kg) (= 0.1 mL/kg of 1:**10,000** soln.)	**2nd (and Subsequent) Doses for IV, IO, or ET* Bolus Administration** (= 0.1 mg/kg) (= 0.1 mL/kg of 1:**1,000** soln.)
10 kg	**0.1 mg** (1 ml of 1:10,000 soln.)	**1 mg** (1 ml of 1:1,000 soln.)
20 kg	**0.2 mg** (2 ml of 1:10,000 soln.)	**2 mg** (2 ml of 1:1,000 soln.)
30 kg	**0.3 mg** (3 ml of 1:10,000 soln.)	**3 mg** (3 ml of 1:1,000 soln.)
Adult Dose	1.0 mg IV (= **SDE**)	*Highly variable* (i.e., *SDE* to *HDE*)

> * **Note**- For simplicity, *we have not indicated the Initial Dose for ET Bolus administration in this Table.* The *initial dose* of **Epinephrine** recommended for **ET bolus administration** of *asystolic or pulseless arrest* is the *SAME* as that recommended for treatment of *symptomatic bradycardia* (= **0.1 mg/kg** = 0.1 mL/kg of 1:1,000 solution).

IV Infusion of Epinephrine

The recommended range for *IV Infusion of Epinephrine* in pediatric patients is *between* **0.1- 1.0 µg/kg/minute**. Preparation for IV infusion may be accomplished as follows:

- Mix [<u>0.6 mg</u> X <u>body weight</u> (kg)] of drug in 100 ml of **diluent** (D5W, NS, or Ringer's lactate). At this concentration:

  - 1 drop/minute = 0.1 µg/kg/minute. *Titrate to effect.*

Weight of Patient	How to Mix *EPINEPHRINE*	*Initial* Rate	*Maximum* Rate*
10 kg	Mix **6 mg** (i.e., 0.6 X 10) in 100 ml	1 drop/minute (= 1 µg/min)	10 drops/min (= 10 µg/min)
20 kg	Mix **12 mg** (i.e., 0.6 X 20) in 100 ml	1 drop/minute (= 2 µg/min)	10 drops/min (= 20 µg/min)
30 kg	Mix **18 mg** (i.e., 0.6 X 30) in 100 ml	1 drop/minute (= 3 µg/min)	10 drops/min (= 30 µg/min)
Adult Dose	1 mg in 250 ml D5W	15-30 drops/minute (= 1-2 µg/min)	*Titrate upward*

* Higher doses may be used if asystole persists and/or the patient fails to respond.

> **Note**- The beauty of preparing pediatric IV infusions using the above parameters (i.e., *mixing* **0.6 mg** of the drug X **body weight** in **kg**- *in 100 ml* of dliluent)- is that the number on the infusion pump (which indicates the number of **ml/hr** infused)- will be *identical* to the number of **drops/minute** !!! Because of the small quantities of drug required for pediatric IV infusions- it is essential to use an *infusion pump* to ensure accuracy.

Atropine

As emphasized in the beginning of this section- **Atropine** should be considered a *second-line* drug (and no more than a *third-line* treatment measure) for management of pediatric bradyarrhythmias. The treatment of choice should always entail focused efforts to ensure that ventilation and oxygenation are adequate. _IF_ despite these efforts pharmacologic therapy *is* still needed for treatment of pediatric bradycardia/asystole- the drug of choice should be **Epinephrine** (and _not_ Atropine).

> The point to emphasize is that Atropine should probably *not* be used to treat pediatric bradycardia- until *after* Epinephrine has been tried *and* adequate oxygenation/ventilation has been assured.

- **IV Dosing of Atropine**- Give **0.02 mg/kg**. May repeat this dose every 5 minutes (if needed)- up to a **total dose** of **1.0 mg** in a <u>child</u>- or up to **2.0 mg** in an <u>adolescent</u> (AHA PALS Text- Pg 6-9).

  Do *not* give less than 0.1 mg in a single dose (regardless of the child's body weight). The *maximal* recommended dose of Atropine for use in pediatric resuscitation is 0.5 mg for a child (or 1.0 mg in an adolescent).

Weight of Patient	Single IV Dose of *Atropine*
10 kg	0.2 mg
20 kg	0.4 mg
30 kg	0.6 mg
Adult Dose	0.5- 1.0 mg

Dopamine

The pharmacologic effects of **Dopamine** are *dose-dependent.* As is the case for adults, infusion of *Epinephrine* may be preferable to Dopamine when there is marked circulatory instability- and/or when hypotension persists *despite* higher infusion rates of Dopamine.

- *At LOW infusion rates* (i.e., **5-10 µg/kg/minute**)- dilates renal and mesenteric blood vessels (so urine output may increase)- but heart rate and BP will usually *not* be affected (i.e., predominant *dopaminergic* effect).

- *At MODERATE infusion rates* (i.e., **10-20 mg/kg/minute**)- increases cardiac output- usually with only a modest effect on peripheral vascular resistance and BP (i.e., *beta-adrenergic* effect prevails).

- *At HIGH infusion rates* (i.e., **>20 µg/kg/minute**)- results in intense peripheral vasoconstriction (as *alpha-adrenergic* effect takes over)- producing a significant increase in peripheral vascular resistance and BP.

Note- Pediatric definitions of dose-related effects with Dopamine infusion differ slightly from those of adults. In general, infusion of Dopamine is begun at a relatively *higher* infusion rate (of **10 µg/kg/minute**) in pediatric patients (AHA PALS Text- Pg 6-13).

IV Infusion Dose of Dopamine

The recommended range for *IV Infusion of Dopamine* in pediatric patients is *between* **10-20 µg/kg/minute**. Preparation for IV infusion may be accomplished as follows:

▪ Mix [6 mg X body weight (kg)] of drug in 100 ml of **diluent** (D5W, NS, or Ringer's lactate). At this concentration:

- 1 drop/minute   =   1.0 µg/kg/minute

   - 10 drops/minute = **10 µg/kg/minute**
        (= usual *initial* rate of infusion)

      - 20 drops/minute   =   20 µg/kg/minute
           (= *maximum* rate of infusion)

Weight of Patient	How to Mix *Dopamine*	*Initial* Rate	*Maximum* Rate
10 kg	Mix **60 mg** (i.e., 6 X 10) in 100 ml	10 drops/minute (= 100 µg/min)	20 drops/min (= 200 µg/min)
20 kg	Mix **120 mg** (i.e., 6 X 20) in 100 ml	10 drops/minute (= 200 µg/min)	20 drops/min (= 400 µg/min)
30 kg	Mix **180 mg** (i.e., 6 X 30) in 100 ml	10 drops/minute (= 300 µg/min)	20 drops/min (= 600 µg/min)
Adult Dose	200 mg in 250 ml D5W	30 drops/minute (= 400 µg/min)	*Titrate upward*

> **Note**- The beauty of preparing pediatric IV infusions using the above parameters (i.e., *mixing 6 mg* of the drug X *body weight* in **kg**- *in 100 ml* of diluent)- is that the number on the infusion pump (which indicates the number of *ml/hr* infused)- will be *identical* to the number of *drops/ minute* (*as well as* to the number of *µg/kg/minute*) !!! Because of the small quantities of drug required for pediatric IV infusions- it is essential to use an *infusion pump* to ensure accuracy.

Lidocaine

Because malignant ventricular arrhythmias are much less commonly seen in association with pediatric cardiopulmonary arrest- *Lidocaine will not be needed in most pediatric codes.*

- ■ ***Bolus Dose****- for **IV** or **IO** administration = **1.0 mg/kg**. Thus, a **10 kg** child should receive a **10 mg** bolus dose of Lidocaine- a 20 kg child should receive 20 mg- and so on.

IV Infusion Dose of Lidocaine

The recommended range for ***IV Infusion of Lidocaine*** in pediatric patients is *between* **20-50 µg/kg/minute**. Preparation for IV infusion may be accomplished as follows:

- ■ Mix <u>120 mg</u> of Lidocaine in 100 ml of D5W (= **1,200 µg/ml** as the *concentration* of drug). At this concentration:

  - 1 drop/kg/minute = 20 µg/kg/minute (*Initial* rate)
  - 2.5 drops/kg/minute = 50 µg/kg/minute (*Maximum* rate).

Weight of Patient	How to Mix *Lidocaine*	*Initial* Rate	*Maximum* Rate
10 kg	120 mg in 100 ml D5W	10 drops/min (= 20 µg/kg/min X 10 kg = 200 µg/min = 0.2 mg/min)	25 drops/min (= 0.5 mg/min)
20 kg	120 mg in 100 ml D5W	20 drops/min (= 400 µg/min = 0.4 mg/min)	50 drops/min (= 1.0 mg/min)
30 kg	120 mg in 100 ml D5W	30 drops/min (= 600 µg/min = 0.6 mg/min)	75 drops/min (= 1.5 mg/min)
Adult Dose	1,000 mg in 250 ml D5W	≈30 drops/min = 2 mg/min	4 mg/min

> **Note**- The beauty of preparing pediatric IV infusions using the above parameters is that the number on the infusion pump (which indicates the number of ***ml/hr*** infused)- will be *identical* to the number of ***drops/minute*** !!! Because of the small quantities of drug required for pediatric IV infusions- it is essential to use an *infusion pump* to ensure accuracy.

Adenosine

As noted at the beginning of this section, the most common tachyarrhythmia to produce hemodynamic instability in *infants* is **PSVT**- which often attains heart rates in excess of 200-250 beats/minute in this age group.

Because of its rapid rate- PSVT may *not* be well tolerated when it occurs in infants or small children. If allowed to persist, infants in particular face a great risk of developing congestive heart failure and/or shock. The *younger* the infant, the *faster* the ventricular rate (especially if >180 beats/minute), and the *longer the duration* of the tachycardia (especially if over 24 hours)- the more likely (*and the sooner*) that heart failure will develop. Clinically then, if the infant does not readily respond to a **vagal maneuver** (i.e., application of an *ice pack* to the face for ≈15 seconds) or pharmacologic therapy (i.e., **Adenosine**)- *and/or* at *any* time develops signs of hemodynamic compromise- *then* **emergency cardioversion** *may be needed.*

In most cases, pharmacologic therapy *can* be used and will be effective for PSVT (so that emergency cardioversion will *not* be needed). **Adenosine** has become the drug of choice in this situation for pediatric patients. Adenosine is extremely effective and appears much *less* likely to produce adverse hemodynamic effects in infants or young children than Verapamil. Even if adverse effects do occur, the exceedingly short half-life of Adenosine (of *less* than 10 seconds) tends to limit their duration.

> **Note**- Although **Verapamil** has been a drug of choice for treatment of PSVT in adults, the drug should be used with extreme caution (if at all) in younger children- especially if they are acutely ill. This is because excessive heart rate slowing, decreased contractility, and profound hypotension (from vasodilatation and negative inotropy) can all occur and produce potentially disastrous consequences in such patients.

- **_IV Dosing of Adenosine_** - Give **0.1 mg/kg** for the *initial* dose. Double this amount (i.e., to **0.2 mg/kg**) if there is no effect. The *maximal* recommended dose of Adenosine for use in pediatric resuscitation is 12 mg.

  As is the case for adults- remember the importance of *rapid* administration of Adenosine (giving the drug *as fast as possible* over 1-3 seconds)- so as to prevent deterioration of drug in the IV tubing. To further facilitate absorption- follow each IV bolus with a fluid flush.

Weight of Patient	Initial IV Dose of *Adenosine*	2nd (*and Subsequent*) Doses
10 kg	1 mg	2 mg
20 kg	2 mg	4 mg
30 kg	3 mg	6 mg
Adult Dose	6 mg	12 mg

Sodium Bicarbonate

Respiratory failure is the most common cause of cardiac arrest in children. As a result, the most important treatment priority in pediatric resuscitation is to improve ventilation- *NOT to administer Sodium Bicarbonate.* Next to oxygen, Epinephrine is the drug of choice for treatment of cardiopulmonary arrest in children. **Sodium Bicarbonate** should be considered *only* if the arrest is prolonged- or if the patient was *known* to have a severe preexisting/underlying metabolic acidosis.

- **_IV (or IO) Dose_**- Give **1 mEq/kg** (where 50 ml of 8.4% solution = 50 mEq).

Weight of Patient	IV (or IO) Dose of SODIUM BICARBONATE
10 kg	10 mEq (1/5 ampule)
20 kg	20 mEq (2/5 ampule)
30 kg	30 mEq (3/5 ampule)
Adult Dose	50-100 mEq (1-2 ampules)

Defibrillation/Cardioversion

VT and V Fib are extremely uncommon terminal events in pediatric arrests. As a result, defibrillation and synchronized cardioversion will only *rarely* be needed during pediatric resuscitation.

- **_Defibrillation Dose_** **2 J**(joules)**/kg** for the *initial* attempt. If unsuccessful- *double* the dose (to **4 J/kg**)- and repeat X 2 (shcoking in *rapid* succession).

- **_Synchronized Cardioversion Dose_** **0.5 J**(joules)**/kg** initially. Increase this amount as needed for subsequent cardioversion attempts.

Weight of Patient	1st *Defib* (2nd - 3rd Shock)	*Cardioversion*
10 kg	20J (then 40J- 40J)	5 J
20 kg	40J (then 80J- 80J)	10 J
30 kg	60J (then 120J- 120J)	15 J
Adult Dose	200J (then 300J- 360J)	*Variable* (≈50-200 J)

Appendix: *Value Added Drug Table*

Oxygen	Dose & Routes of Administration	Comments
Indications - *Suspected* hypoxemia of any cause (including cardiopulmonary arrest, acute ischemic chest pain, Acute MI, etc.).	**Nasal Canula**- 24-40% oxygen can be delivered with flow rates of 6L/min. **Face Mask/Pocket Mask**- up to 50% oxygen can be delivered with flow rates of 10L/min. **Venturi Mask**- offers a decided advantage over the nasal canula and face mask in that *fixed* oxygen rates (of 24%, 28%, 35%, and 40%) may be delivered- a particularly helpful feature for pts with chronic obstructive pulmonary disease and a history of CO_2 retention. **Non-Rebreathing Oxygen Mask**- superior device for delivering high oxygen concentrations (of up to 90%).	Oxygen is one of the truly *essential* drugs. It should *never* be withheld in an emergency situation for fear of suppressing a pt's respiratory drive. This simply *won't* happen with numerous caregivers at the bedside. Use 100% F_{IO2} during resuscitation! Oxygen toxicity may become a problem with *continual* delivery of high oxygen concentration ($F_{IO2} \geq 50\%$)- when it is given for a *prolonged* period of time (i.e., *more* than 3 days). It is *not* a problem with short term delivery of 100% oxygen during the period of cardiopulmonary resuscitation.

(See also pages 24, 31-32, 44, 102, 107-109, 119-120, 128, 132-133, 136-141P)

Epinephrine	Dose & Routes of Administration	Comments

Indications
 	
- V Fib or pulseless VT
- Asystole
- EMD/PEA
 	
- Use of Epinephrine (by IV infusion) may also be considered for treatment of hemodynamically significant bradyarrhythmias that have *not* responded to Atropine.
	Initial IV Dose- **1.0 mg** by IV bolus = **SDE** (= 10 ml of a 1:10,000 soln).
	
	Subsequent IV Dosing- Epinephrine should be repeated every **3-5 minutes** in cardiac arrest. After the initial **SDE** (= 1 mg) IV dose- one may either *continue* with 1 mg IV doses- or chose between *several **HDE** alternatives* :
	
	- Administration
	    of **2-5 mg** IV boluses-
	
	    - O R -
	
	- *escalating*
	    1- 3- 5 mg IV boluses-
	
	    - O R -
	
	- dosing at **0.1 mg/kg** as an
	    IV bolus.
	
	ET Route- *recommended for use if IV access is unavailable.* Instill 2-2.5 times the IV dose (i.e., **2-2.5 mg** of 1:10,000 soln.) down the ET tube- and follow with several forceful insufflations of the Ambu bag.
		The alpha-adrenergic (= vasoconstrictor) effect of Epinephrine is the most important one in cardiac arrest (because this effect increases aortic diastolic pressure). Blood flow to coronary arteries is favored, and there is preferential shunting of blood from the external to the internal carotid artery.
		
		The *"optimal dose"* of Epinephrine remains unknown. AHA Guidelines clearly allow for *flexibility* in Epinephrine dosing by stating that *"use of HDE can neither be recommended nor discouraged"* (AHA Text- Pg 7-4).
		
		Use of HDE for pts with refractory V Fib may increase the likelihood of ROSC (return of spontaneous circulation). Unfortunately- because of the longer time until discovery and treatment of many of these pts, there is also a greater chance of permanent neurologic sequelae. Judgement is therefore needed in deciding whether or not to use **HDE**- and if so, under what circumstances.
		
		The effect of an IV bolus of Epinephrine peaks in 2-3 minutes (which is the reason AHA Guidelines now allow for repetition of each bolus as often as every 3 minutes for as long as the pt remains in cardiac arrest).

Epinephrine
(Continued)

Indications

Dose & Routes of Administration	Comments
IV Infusion of Epinephrine - may be administered in both standard and high dose form: - **Standard Dosing (= SDE)**- Mix **1 mg** of a **1:10,000** soln. of Epinephrine in **250 ml** of D5W- and *begin* the infusion @ **15-30 drops/min** (=1-2 µg/min). Titrate the rate of infusion upward as needed. - **High-Dose Epinephrine (= HDE)**- Mix **50 mg** of a **1:1,000** soln. of Epinephrine in **250 ml** of D5W- and *begin* the infusion @ **30-60 drops/min** (=100-200 µg/min). Titrate the rate of infusion upward as needed. NOTE- An IV infusion rate of **200 µg/min** will deliver 1,000 µg = **1 mg** of Epinephrine every **5 min**- *which is* (= 200 X 5 = 1,000 µg)- *comparable to an SDE dose of Epinephrine* !	When Epinephrine is used to treat pts who are *not* in cardiac arrest (i.e., for treatment of symptomatic bradycardia with a pulse)- a *lower dose* of drug (i.e., SDE) should be used- and the Epinephrine should be administered by *continuous* **IV infusion** instead of by IV bolus. This is because if adverse effects do occur- "*you can't take the effect of a bolus back*". Use of Epinephrine by continuous IV infusion allows *moment-to-moment* titration of dose. Compared to Dopamine- Epinephrine may be preferable for use as a *pressor* agent in the treatment of bradycardia with more severe hemodynamic impairment.

Lidocaine	Dose & Routes of Administration	Comments
Indications - Drug of choice for *refractory V Fib* and acute treatment of ventricular ectopy (*PVCs, VT*)- when such treatment is indicated. - Appropriate for treatment of *wide-complex* tachycardias of unknown etiology (which statistically are most likely to be VT).	**IV Bolus** (Treatment of PVCs/VT)- Give **1.0-1.5 mg/kg** (= 50-150 mg) as an *initial* bolus. Repeat boluses of ≈50-75 mg may be given every 5-10 minutes up to a total of ≈3 mg/kg (i.e., ≈225 mg). - - - - - - - - - - - - - - - **IV Infusion**- Mix **1g** in **250 ml** of D5W- and begin drip @ **30 drops/min (= 2 mg/min)**. - The usual *range* of IV infusion = 0.5-4.0 mg/min (although most pts are adequately treated at a rate of between 1-2 mg/minute). - - - - - - - - - - - - - - - **IV Bolus** (Treatment of V Fib)- Give **1.0-1.5 mg/kg** (= 50-150 mg) as an *initial* bolus. May repeat in 3-5 minutes- *although a single IV dose of **1.5 mg/kg**) is acceptable in cardiac arrest. NOTE- IV infusion is *not* necessarily needed while the pt remains in V Fib! **ET Tube**- Use 2 to 2.5 times the IV dose (=100-150 mg) to obtain equivalent blood levels as with IV administration.	Remember to start a *prophylactic IV* infusion of Lidocaine immediately after converting a pt out of V Fib (in the hope of preventing recurrence of V Fib). For pts who only received IV boluses during cardiac arrest- rebolus of the drug may be needed prior to starting the IV infusion. In the *spontaneously beating heart*, the half-life of Lidocaine is short (i.e., ≈10 minutes). As a result, an IV infusion of the drug *must* be started *within* 5-10 minutes of giving an IV bolus (or the effect of the bolus will be dissipated). However, because clearance of Lidocaine is markedly impaired during cardiac arrest- one need *not* necessarily begin the IV infusion until after the pt is converted out of V Fib. Not every PVC need be eliminated for Lidocaine to exert a protective effect. Maintenance of a therapeutic serum level of Lidocaine may be all that is needed to protect against development of VT/V Fib- even if "breakthrough" PVCs are still occurring.

Bretylium	Dose & Routes of Administration	Comments
Indications	**IV Bolus** *(for Refractory V Fib)*- 5 mg/kg initially (or a single **500 mg** bolus = **1 amp**). Defibrillate ≈1 min later. If V Fib persists, a **2nd dose** (of 10 mg/kg or ≈1-2 amps) may be given 5 min later. This 10 mg/kg dose may be repeated *twice* at 5-30 min intervals (up to a total loading dose of 30-35 mg/kg).	Bretylium has been used less in recent years for a number of reasons:
- Drug of 2nd choice for *refractory V Fib* (after Lidocaine).		- The drug has *not* been shown to be superior to Lidocaine for treatment of V Fib.
- 3rd-line agent for acute treatment of PVCs/VT.		- Lidocaine appears less likely to produce adverse hemodynamic effects during CPR.
	- Be sure to circulate the drug with CPR (for ≈1-2 min) after each administration- and then *defibrillate* again.	- Most clinicians are more familiar (and comfortable) with the use of Lidocaine.
NOTE- The sympathomimetic effects of Bretylium may on some occasions initially aggravate ventricular arrhythmias- which is why use of the drug is now generally reserved for those pts who are truly symptomatic from their arrhythmia.	**IV Infusion**- Mix **1g** in **250 ml** of D5W- and begin drip @ **15-30 drops/min (=1-2 mg/min)**.	Although the onset of action of Bretylium is usually within a few minutes when treating V Fib- its onset may sometimes be *delayed* for up to 2-20 minutes (especially when the rhythm is VT).
	IV Loading Infusion *(for VT)*- Dilute **500 mg** (≈1 amp) in 50 ml of D5W, and infuse over ≈10 minutes (i.e., giving a dose of ≈5-10 mg/kg). May repeat IV loading of another 5-10 mg/kg (i.e.- ≈500 mg) in 10-30 minutes (again infused over ≈10 min).	The duration of action of a Bretylium bolus is 2-6 hrs. Use of a **Bretylium IV infusion** (@ 1-2 mg/min) may help to maintain the effect of the drug- especially for pts with *refractory V Fib* who only responded after Bretylium was added.
		Hypotension is the most common (and limiting) side effect of IV maintenance infusion with Bretylium.

PROCAINAMIDE

(See also pages 34, 44, 67, 80, 90, 94)

Procainamide	Dose & Routes of Administration	Comments
Indications	**IV Loading:** Give in increments of 100 mg *slowly* over a 5 minute period (@ ≈20 mg/min)- *until* one or more of the following *end points* are reached:	Hypotension is exacerbated with more rapid IV infusion of Procainamide (i.e., @ >30 mg/min). Hypotension is the major limiting factor in IV use of this drug.
- Drug of 2nd choice (after Lidocaine) for acute treatment of ventricular ectopy (PVCs, VT).	- the arrhythmia is suppressed - hypotension occurs - the QRS widens by ≥50% - a total loading dose of **17 mg/ kg** has been given (which comes out to ≈1,000 mg for the *average-sized* adult).	Procainamide is available in both oral and IV forms- which is a decided advantage for pts in need of long-term maintenance therapy.
- Treatment of A Fib/Flutter (similar action as Quinidine that may help in conversion of A Fib/Flutter to normal sinus rhythm).		
- *Possibly* for refractory V Fib (although *not* nearly as effective as Lidocaine and Bretylium for this indication).	**Alternative IV Loading Regimen-** Mix ≈500-1,000 mg of drug in 100 ml of D5W- and infuse this over 30-60 minutes (keeping in mind the *end points* of infusion noted above).	Even when IV Procainamide does not convert a pt out of sustained VT- it may slow the *rate* of the VT (which may allow the pt to tolerate the arrhythmia better).
- May be invaluable in the treatment of *wide-complex tachycardia* of uncertain etiology (since this drug may effectively treat *both* VT and PSVT- *as well as* rapid A Fib with WPW).	**IV Infusion**- Mix **1g** in **250 ml** of D5W- and begin drip @ **30 drops/ min (=2 mg/min).**	Procainamide works in the treatment of rapid A Fib with WPW by slowing conduction in the *antegrade* direction down the accessory pathway.
	- Use of an **IV infusion** may be considered to *maintain* the drug's effect following IV loading.	Procainamide should *not* be used for treatment of *Torsade de Pointes* (since use of this drug may further prolong the QT interval- and therefore exacerbate the arrhythmia).
	- Usual *range* of infusion = 1-4 mg/min.	

MAGNESIUM

(See also pages 30, 81, 90, 94, 104)

Magnesium	Dose & Routes of Administration	Comments
Indications **Torsade de Pointes**- for which Magnesium is clearly the medical treatment of choice! **Refractory VT/V Fib**- for which the mechanism of action of the drug is unclear. However, *empiric* use of Magnesium may be helpful in some pts- *even when serum levels are normal* (especially when standard measures have failed). - **Acute MI/PVCs/SVTs** (including PSVT, MAT, and A Fib)- use is controversial, although the drug *may* be helpful. - **Suspected body depletion of Magnesium**- regardless of serum levels, *intracellular* Magnesium deficiency is likely in pts who manifest other electrolyte disturbances (i.e., hyponatremia, hypokalemia, hypocalcemia, and hypophosphatemia). Strong consideration should be given to *empiric* administration of 1-4 g over several hours in such pts.	**For V Fib**- Give **1-2 g IV** of Magnesium Sulfate (= 2-4 ml of a 50% soln.)- by **IV push**. May repeat in 1-2 minutes if no response. **For VT or Torsade de Pointes**- Give **1-2 g IV** of Magnesium Sulfate (= 2-4 ml of a 50% soln.)- over 1-2 minutes. May repeat in a few minutes if no response. Significantly higher doses (of up to 5-10 g) are sometimes needed for treatment of Torsade. **For *Less Urgent* Treatment Situations** (i.e. treatment of PVCs and/or Acute MI)- consider *more gradual* IV infusion of ≈1-2 g of Magnesium Sulfate over ≥20 minutes. Alternatively, may add the drug to the pt's IV fluids and infuse it over a period of hours (i.e., at a rate of between ≈0.5-1 g/hour for up to 24 hrs). - - - - - - - - - - - - - - - - - Give *lower* doses of Magnesium to pts with renal failure.	Dosing of Magnesium is largely *empiric*! The exact amount of drug required in a given clinical situation is simply *not* known! Clearly the drug needs to be given *faster* for life threatening arrhythmias (i.e., by IV push for V Fib- or over 1-2 minutes for VT). It may be given by more gradual IV infusion for less urgent clinical situations (such as for treatment of PVCs and/or Acute MI). Comfort can be taken in the fact that with rare exceptions- IV administration of Magnesium (*even in large doses!*) is surprisingly free of adverse effects. Most often nothing more is seen than transient flushing, slight hypotension or transient bradycardia- all of which usually resolve with *slowing* of the rate of IV infusion. Ready availability of **Calcium Chloride** is suggested as a "safeguard" when administering Magnesium- in the rare event that marked hypotension or asystole is produced.

Atropine	Dose & Routes of Administration	Comments
Indications - Hemodynamically significant bradyarrhythmias (including **"relative bradycardia"**)- for which Atropine remains the pharmacologic intervention of choice (AHA Text- Pg 1-30). - Asystole - PEA - Atropine is most likely to work when used to treat bradycardia in the early hours of acute *inferior* infarction (when increased parasympathetic tone is most likely to be at least partially responsible for the reduction in heart rate). - Caution is advised when using Atropine in the setting of Acute MI to treat 2° or 3° AV block with QRS widening. Use of cardiac pacing may be preferable in this situation.	**IV Bolus:** - *Not in Cardiac Arrest*- Give **0.5-1.0 mg IV**; may repeat every 3-5 minutes- *if/as needed* (up to a total dose of 2-3 mg). - *In Bradyasystolic Arrest*- Give **1.0 mg IV** at a time; may repeat every 3-5 minutes- *if/as needed* (up to a total dose of **0.04 mg/kg** or ≈3 mg). ---------- **ET Tube**- 1-2 mg at a time (diluted in 10 ml of normal saline or sterile H₂O)- and followed by several forceful insufflations of the Ambu bag.	Although 2 mg will be the *full atropinization dose* for many pts- up to **0.04 mg/kg** (i.e, *up to ≈3 mg* in an *average-sized* adult) may occasionally be needed to obtain maximal effect. In general, lower doses of Atropine (i.e., **0.5 mg IV**) are preferred for *initial* treatment of pts with bradycardia who are *not* in cardiac arrest- especially if symptoms are less severe. Higher doses (i.e., **1 mg** at a time) may be tried in pts with more severe symptoms- and/or for those who fail to respond to a 0.5 mg dose. Use of a maximal dose of Atropine (i.e., ≈3 mg) is most often *reserved* for treatment of pts with bradyasystolic cardiac arrest. AHA Guidelines allow for more frequent dosing of Atropine (*as often as every 1-3 minutes!*) for pts with *marked* hemodynamic compromise from bradycardia. Use of Atropine is *not benign!* The drug may unmask previously undetected excess sympathetic tone- and thereby precipitate ventricular tachyarrhythmias. On rare occasions, the drug may also produce paradoxical slowing of the ventricular response if given to pts with more advanced AV block. For these reasons- Atropine should *only* be used to treat pts with hemodynamically significant bradyarrhythmias.

(See also pages 45, 128, 143P)

Dopamine	Dose & Routes of Administration	Comments
Indications - Hemodynamically significant bradyarrhythmias that have *not* responded to Atropine (when cardiac pacing is unavailable) - Cardiogenic shock NOTE- Dopamine is generally accepted as the initial pressor agent of choice for treatment of hemodynamically significant bradycardia when symptoms are not too severe. With more profound hypotension, IV infusion of Epinephrine may be preferred.	**IV Infusion**- Mix 1 amp (**200 mg**) in **250 ml** of D5W- and begin drip @ **15-30 drops/min** (= 2-5 µg/kg/ minute). Titrate to clinical response. NOTE- moderate to high infusion rates of Dopamine produce an effect that resembles Epinephrine (and may be used to maintain coronary perfusion in the arrested heart). As the infusion rate is increased even further (i.e., to ≈15-20 µg/kg/min), the drug becomes progressively more like Norepinephrine (i.e., a pure vasoconstrictor).	- At *LOW infusion rates* (i.e., 1-2 µg/kg/min- and perhaps up to 5 µg/kg/min)- dilates renal and mesenteric blood vessels (so urine output may increase)- but heart rate and BP will usually *not* be affected (i.e., predominant *dopaminergic effect*). - At *MODERATE infusion rates* (i.e., 2-10 µg/kg/min)- increases cardiac output- usually with only a modest effect on peripheral vascular resistance and BP (i.e., *beta-adrenergic effect prevails*). - At *HIGH infusion rates* (i.e., >10 µg/kg/min)- results in intense peripheral vasoconstriction (as *alpha-adrenergic* effect takes over)- producing a significant increase in peripheral vascular resistance and BP. NOTE- Despite the above general guidelines for dose-dependent effects of Dopamine, there is still some patient-to-patient variability in dosing. Thus, some pts may manifest predominant alpha-adrenergic effects at relatively low infusion rates- whereas in others, beta-adrenergic effects may still predominate at high infusion rates. Individualization of dosing is therefore essential.

Morphine	Dose & Routes of Administration	Comments
Indications - Acute ischemic chest pain - Pulmonary edema - - - - - - - - - - **Mechanism**- Morphine markedly increases venous capacitance (and thus reduces preload), produces mild arterial vasodilatation (thus lowering afterload to a small degree), and reduces acute ischemic chest pain and the anxiety of acute air hunger.	**IV Bolus**- Give in small (i.e., **1-3 mg**) *incremental* **IV doses**. Higher doses (i.e., of 3-5 mg) may be used if the drug is tolerated and symptoms are severe. May repeat IV dosing every 5-30 minutes (as needed).	Although IV nitroglycerin is the drug of choice for acute ischemic chest pain- incremental dosing with Morphine is still an extremely useful adjunct when symptoms are severe and persistent. Morphine may cause oversedation and/or *respiratory depression* (which *is* reversible with 0.4-0.8 mg IV **Naloxone**). Morphine may also occasionally cause bradycardia or hypotension (which is usually easily treated by placing pt in Trendelenburg position, fluids- and if needed, Atropine). Morphine remains a treatment of choice for acute pulmonary edema. The drug reduces preload and afterload- as well as attenuating the anxiety and air hunger inherent with pulmonary edema.

(See also pages 64, 73-74, 89, 99-102, 146P)

Verapamil	Dose & Routes of Administration	Comments
Indications	**IV Dosing**- Begin with a dose of **2.5-5 mg IV** (to be given over a 1-2 min period). Give the drug *slower* (i.e., over 3-4 min) in the elderly or in those with borderline BP.	Combining small doses of Verapamil/Diltiazem with IV Digoxin- may produce a *synergistic* effect when treating rapid A Fib/Flutter.
PSVT- >90% success rate in converting to sinus rhythm.	- May give up to 5-10 mg in a dose (and repeat several times in 15-30 min if/as needed)- up to a total dose of ≈30 mg.	Pretreatment with **Calcium Chloride** (giving 500-1,000 mg IV over a 5-10 min period) minimizes the hypotensive response of Verapamil/Diltiazem *without* affecting its antiarrhythmic efficacy.
MAT- treatment of choice when rate control is needed.	**Oral Dosing**: 120-480 mg daily, divided into three equal doses (or given less often if sustained release preparations are used).	*Do not* use Verapamil/Diltiazem to treat *wide-complex* tachycardias (WCTs) of uncertain etiology!
Atrial Fib/Flutter- effectively slows ventricular response.		*Do not* use Verapamil/Diltiazem to treat rapid A Fib with WPW.
NOTE- Use of either Verapamil or Diltiazem is more effective than Digoxin for rate control of A Fib/Flutter in *both* the acute and chronic setting.		*Do not* use Verapamil/Diltiazem within 30 minutes of using an IV β-blocker.
		Should calcium channel blocker toxicity develop (i.e., significant bradycardia/asystole)- in response to administration of Verapamil or Diltiazem- the treatment of choice is with **Calcium Chloride** (page 170).

Adenosine	Dose & Routes of Administration	Comments
Indications **PSVT** (and other *reentry* tachyarrhythmias including PSVT associated with WPW). Adenosine is now the drug of 1st choice for emergency treatment of PSVT. As a *diagnostic maneuver* (i.e., "chemical Valsalva") in pts with SVT of *uncertain* etiology. Adenosine will probably convert the rhythm if it is a reentry tachycardia. Otherwise, it will probably produce *transient slowing* (which will hopefully enable atrial activity to be seen- so as to allow the correct diagnosis to be made). --- **Caution**- Adenosine is *not* a completely benign agent. We therefore feel that the drug should *not* be given if the rhythm is *known* to be VT.	**IV Bolus**- initially give **6 mg** by **IV push**. If no response after 1-2 min, give **12 mg** by IV push- which may be repeated a final time 1-2 min later (for a **total dose** of 6 + 12 + 12 = **30 mg**). --- - Higher than usual doses of Adenosine may be needed for pts receiving Theophylline. - Lower than usual doses may be needed for cardiac transplant recipients and for pts on Persantine/Tegretol. - Caution is advised in the use of Adenosine in pts with sick sinus syndrome and/or a history of AV conduction defects.	Be sure to give Adenosine by **IV push** (i.e., injecting the drug *as fast as possible* over 1-3 seconds!)- and follow each dose with a **saline flush** (of ≈20 ml of fluid). Otherwise the drug will deteriorate *within* the IV tubing. The half-life of Adenosine is exceedingly short (i.e., *less than* 10 seconds!). As a result, little time is needed to find out if the drug will work- and any adverse effects that are produced are likely to be extremely short-lived. Realize however that a longer-acting agent may need to be added to prevent recurrence of PSVT. Adverse effects that may be seen include facial flushing, cough/dyspnea, chest pain, and bradycardia. The drug should *not* be given to pts with frank bronchospasm or asthma. Because of its short half-life, Adenosine is in general *unlikely* to cause deterioration of a *wide-complex tachycardia*- even if the drug is inadvertently given to a pt who turns out to have VT.

(See also pages 63-67, 76, 99-102)

Diltiazem	Dose & Routes of Administration	Comments
Indications **PSVT**- >90% success rate in converting to sinus rhythm. **MAT**- treatment of choice when rate control is needed. **Atrial Fib/Flutter**- effectively slows ventricular response. --- NOTE- Use of either Verapamil or Diltiazem is more effective than Digoxin for rate control of A Fib/Flutter in *both* the acute and chronic setting.	**IV Bolus:** - For the average-sized adult, begin with an *initial* **IV bolus of 20 mg** (or 0.25 mg/kg)- given over a 2 minute period. - If the desired response is *not* obtained within 15 minutes- may increase the dose with a **2nd IV bolus of 25 mg** (or 0.35 mg/kg). Dosing for any subsequent boluses should be individualized. --- - Remember that the doses cited above are for an *average-sized* adult! *Smaller doses* (i.e., of ≈10-15 mg) should be given to pts of light body weight. **IV Infusion**- Mix **250 mg** of Diltiazem in **250 ml** of diluant (to make a **concentration** of 1,000 mg in 1,000 ml = **1 mg/ml**). - Begin infusion at **10 mg/hr** (= 10 drops/minute). - Usual rate of infusion is between **10-15 mg/hr** (although some pts only need 5 mg/hr). --- **Oral Dosing**- 90-360 mg daily, divided into three or four equal doses (or given less often if sustained release preparations are used).	Clinical effects from an IV bolus of Diltiazem usually *begin* within 3 minutes- *peak* by 7 minutes- and *last* for 1-3 hours (after which an IV infusion may be used if needed to provide continued rate control). Characteristics of Diltiazem are generally quite similar to those of Verapamil (*See Comments under Verapamil on page 161*). However, Diltiazem does appear to offer several advantages: - availability of an approved formulation for use as continuous IV infusion (which facilitates dose titration and allows *maintenance* of antiarrhythmic effect). - less hypotension/LV depression than IV Verapamil. - minimal effect on serum Digoxin levels (whereas Verapamil may increase the serum Digoxin level by up to 50%). Perhaps the clinical niche for IV Diltiazem is treatment of rapid A Fib/Flutter- in that continuous IV infusion allows for *continued* rate control (and thereby avoids the need for repeated IV bolus dosing of Digoxin and Verapamil).

Propranolol	Dose & Routes of Administration	Comments
Indications	**IV Dose**: Give **0.5-1.0 mg** by *slow* IV (i.e., over a 5 minute period). May repeat as needed (up to a *total* dose of ≈3-5 mg).	Although *not* commonly used in the setting of cardiac arrest- there clearly are times when an IV β-blocker is the *only* medication likely to successfully resuscitate the pt.
Emergency care situations in which **IV β-Blockers** are most likely to be helpful include:		
- Treatment of supraventricular or ventricular arrhythmias that occur in association with (and/or because of) excessive *sympathetic* tone (i.e., in pts with acute *anterior* MI and/or when hypertension or tachycardia *precede* the arrest).	NOTE- Because of ease of administration and familiarity with its use- **Propranolol** is the IV β-blocker most commonly selected for treatment of pts in cardiac arrest. Alternatively, other β-blockers could be used instead:	The mechanism of action of β-blockers appears to be *multifactorial* (due to a *combination* of antiarrhythmic effect, blocking of catecholamine stimulation, reduced myocardial contractility, decreased oxygen consumption, and lowering of BP).
- Cardiac arrest from *cocaine* (or *amphetamine*) overdose.	- **Atenolol**- 5 mg IV over 5 minutes; may repeat in 10 min.	**Caution**- IV β-blockers should *not* be given in close proximity to either IV Verapamil or IV Diltiazem (as doing so may cause marked bradycardia- or even asystole!).
- Severe *psychogenic* stress in the prearrest period.	- **Metoprolol**- 5 mg IV over 2 to 5 minutes; may repeat X 2 every 5 min.	
- Antecedent *ischemia* (i.e., ST segment depression) *prior* to the arrest.	- **Esmolol**- *dosing is listed on page 166.*	**Contraindications**- acute bronchospasm, heart failure, and/or intraventricular conduction disturbances.
- *Empiric* use in the treatment of cardiac arrest when other (more standard) measures have failed.		
- In the treatment of *acute MI*- for which IV β-Blockers have been shown to reduce mortality (especially when used *within* the first 24 hrs after onset of symptoms).		

(See also pages 65, 75, 100)

Digoxin	Dose & Routes of Administration	Comments
Indications **Rapid A Fib/Flutter-** Dig may help with *rate control* (especially if the pt is in heart failure). **PSVT-** although *other* drugs (i.e., Adenosine, Verapamil, Diltiazem) work faster and are more effective in the acute setting. NOTE- Indications for Digoxin are limited in the acute care setting. While we emphasize that use of this drug *is* still appropriate for acute treatment of A Fib/Flutter- *other* drugs (i.e., Diltiazem, Verapamil, and/or β-blockers) may be preferable (and more effective) for this indication. If Digoxin is selected for treatment, keep in mind that the addition of a second rate-slowing agent may be needed if Digoxin alone fails to adequately control the ventricular response.	**IV Digoxin Dosing:** - If the pt has *not* previously been digitalized, consider **IV loading** with an *initial* dose of **0.25-0.5 mg.** - This may be followed with **0.125-0.25 mg IV increments** given every 2-6 hrs (until a *total* loading dose of 0.75-1.5 mg has been administered over the first 24 hrs). - The next day, the daily *maintenance* dose may be started. **Oral Digoxin Dosing:** - The daily *oral* maintenance dose of Digoxin for *most* adults under 60 yrs old (who have normal renal function)- is **0.25 mg/day.** - *Lower* doses (**0.125 mg daily**- or every *other* day) are recommended for **older pts** (and/or in those with impaired renal function). - If there is less clinical urgency, a pt may be slowly (and *safely*) loaded with Digoxin over a period of ≈1-2 weeks- simply by starting them on their expected daily dose. The pt and serum digoxin level should be checked at the end of this time.	Digoxin slows heart rate by increasing *vagal* (= parasympathetic) tone. It is therefore likely to be *less* effective in situations in which catecholamines (and sympathetic tone) are increased (i.e., exercise, stress, acute illness)- which explains why *other* rate-slowing agents (i.e., Verapamil, Diltiazem, β-blockers) may be more effective in such cases. Digoxin may exert a *synergistic* (1 + 1 = 5) effect when used in small doses *in conjunction* with other rate-slowing drugs. Effects of IV Digoxin begin more rapidly than is generally appreciated (i.e., onset of action is often *within* 5-10 minutes- and certainly within 30-60 minutes). The most commonly used oral form of Digoxin (= **Lanoxin**) is *only* 65-70% bioavailable (so that an oral dose of 0.325-0.35 mg is comparable to an IV dose of ≈0.25 mg). The *half-life* of Digoxin is between **36 hours** (in a healthy, young adult)- and **5 days** (in an elderly pt with severe renal impairment). It may therefore take a pt with renal failure who presents with a toxic serum Digoxin level of 4.0 ng/ml about 4-5 days after stopping the drug for the Digoxin level to decrease by *half* (i.e., to ≈2.0 ng/ml)- and another few days for the level to fall back into the therapeutic range.

Esmolol	Dose & Routes of Administration	Comments
Indications	**IV Dosing:**	Esmolol is a *cardioselective β-blocking* agent with a *rapid* onset and *short* duration of action. Pharmacologic effects usually dissipate within 15-30 minutes after stopping the drug.
- Similar to those for Propranolol (*See description for Propranolol on page 164 in this Table*).	- Administer an *initial IV loading dose* (of **250-500 µg/kg**) over a 1 minute period.	
	- Follow with a 4 minute infusion @ **25-50 µg/kg/min.**	Contraindications are similar to those for IV Propranolol (although Esmolol's cardioselectivity may make it somewhat less likely to precipitate bronchospasm in susceptible pts).
	- If desired response is not obtained, titrate the rate of infusion *upward* by **25-50 µg/kg/min** at 5-10 minute intervals (up to a *maximal* dose of 300 µg/kg/min).	Drawbacks of IV Esmolol are the frequency of *hypotension* (which occurs in up to 50% of pts)- and *complexity* of the dosing regimen.
	- May then begin oral antiarrhythmic (and taper Esmolol).	
	- It is generally best *not* to exceed 200 µg/minute (as doing so greatly increases the incidence of hypotension).	**Caution-** IV β-blockers should *not* be given in close proximity to either IV Verapamil or IV Diltiazem (as doing so may cause marked bradycardia- or even asystole!).

Amiodarone	Dose & Routes of Administration	Comments
Indications **In Cardiac Arrest**- refractory V Fib. **In Emergency Cardiac Care**- life-threatening ventricular arrhythmias *not* responsive to other therapy: selected pts with refractory supraventriculararrhythmias /tachyarrhythmias associatd with WPW.	- Until results from additional studies become available, dosing recommendations for Amiodarone in the setting of cardiac arrest will be largely *empiric*. The Medical Letter recommends the following regimen (Vol 37: 114, 1995): - Consider rapid **IV loading** of **150 mg** over a 10-minute period. May repeat (one or more times) for recurrent VT/V Fib. - May follow with slow IV infusion of 1 mg/min (= 60 mg/hour) for the next 6 hours- which may then be followed by *slower* IV maintenance infusion (of **0.5 mg/min** = 30 mg/hour) over the next 1-4 days.	IV Amiodarone has recently been approved for general use in this country. However, the drug is *not* yet included in AHA ACLS Guidelines! In the future, IV Amiodarone may assume a useful role in the treatment of pts with *refractory* VT/V Fib- especially for the pt who goes in and out of these rhythms! Use of *oral* Amiodarone is associated with *numerous* side effects- and is therefore best left to a specialist- and in arrhythmia management.

Aminophylline	Dose & Routes of Administration	Comments
Indications - May be considered for *brady-asystolic arrest* (or *severe* hemodynamically significant bradycardia) that is *refractory* to standard measures.	**IV Dose**- Give **250 mg IV** over a 1-2 minute period; may repeat.	Aminophylline is *not yet* included in AHA ACLS Guidelines ! Postulated mechanism relates to fact that endogenously released Adenosine is a naturally occurring mediator of bradyasystolic arrest and severe ischemic states- and that Aminophylline is a *competitive antagonist* of Adenosine. Although use of Aminophylline for treatment of bradyasystolic arrest is clearly controversial- small studies suggest that this drug may restore a rhythm in *selected* pts who fail to respond to Atropine, Epinephrine and pacing. Practically speaking- there may be little to lose in such situations (i.e., *"You can't be deader than dead"*)- so that empiric trial of Aminophylline may not be unreasonable if standard measures have not been successful.

Sodium Bicarbonate	Dose & Routes of Administration	Comments
Indications - Indications are limited in the setting of cardiac arrest to *severe* metabolic acidosis that persists *beyond* the initial phase (i.e., beyond the first 5-15 minutes) - and/or cardiac arrest in a pt *known* to have a severe *pre-existing* metabolic acidosis *prior* to the arrest- - *IF* any Bicarb is indicated at all . . . . NOTE- Severe special resuscitation situations do exist in which use of Bicarb is both appropriate and *likely* to be helpful. They include: - Hyperkalemia. - Tricyclic antidepressant overdose (aiming to keep serum pH between 7.45-7.55). - Phenobarbital overdose (aiming to alkalinize the urine). - After the code is over (if severe metabolic acidosis persists).	*IF* Sodium Bicarbonate is felt to be indicated at all- then an *initial dose* of **1 mEq/kg** (=1-1.5 amps) has been recommended. No more than *half* this amount should be given every 10 minutes. In the postresuscitation phase, ABGs should guide therapy. NOTE- If you do chose to administer Bicarb empirically in cardiac arrest- it may be advisable *not* to give the drug for the initial 5-10 minutes of the arrest (since it usually takes *at least* this long to develop a metabolic acidosis in cardiac arrest). - It should be emphasized that the initial cause of acidosis in cardiac arrest is *hypoventilation* (that is best corrected by improving ventilation- and *not* by giving Bicarb).	Remember that *"good CPR is the best buffer therapy."* (AHA Text- Pg 7-15). Standard ABG studies in cardiac arrest *cannot* be relied upon (because they do *not* accurately reflect the true state of *intracellular* homeostasis). --- Drawbacks of administering Sodium Bicarbonate to pts in cardiac arrest include that: - the drug has *not* been shown to improve survival. - the principal cause of acidosis during the *early* minutes of cardiac arrest (i.e., *hypoventilation*) is *not* corrected by Bicarb administration. - the degree of *intracellular* acidosis paradoxically *worsens* (despite "improvement" of ABG values)! - other significant *adverse effects* may occur (including *iatrogenic* alkalosis, hyperosmolality, hypokalemia, sodium overload, impaired oxygen delivery to tissues, seizures, arrhythmias- and impaired left ventricular function from the negative inotropic effect of excess CO_2).

Calcium Chloride	Dose & Routes of Administration	Comments
Indications Limited in the acute care setting to 4 clinical situations: 1. *Hypocalcemia.* 2. *Hyperkalemia.* 3. As *pre-treatment* prior to giving Verapamil/Diltiazem. 4. Treatment of *calcium channel blocker toxicity* (i.e., if marked bradycardia or asystole occurs following use of Verapamil/Diltiazem. NOTE: Caclium is *no longer* indicated for treatment of EMD/asystole!	**IV Bolus**- Give **500-1,000 mg** (5-10 ml) by *slow IV* (over 5-10 minutes). May repeat every 10 minutes if needed (up to 2-4 g). NOTE: Infusion of calcium as *pre-treatment* minimizes the hypotensive response of Verapamil/ Diltiazem. Diltiazem without diminishing their efficacy in converting/controlling the ventricular response of supraventricular tachyarrhythmias. Calcium preinfusion might be considered particularly for pts with borderline hemodynamic status (i.e., systolic BP ≤100) in association with their tachyarrhythmia.	The 10% solution of Calcium Chloride contains 1,000 mg (= 13.6 mEq) of calcium per 10 ml syringe. Don't forget that the "antidote" of calcium channel blocker toxicity is *calcium.* Although **Calcium Chloride** is clearly the most commonly used IV form of this cation- *other* preparations are available (i.e., **Calcium Gluconate**). These other preparations contain *different* amounts of elemental calcium !!!

Isoproterenol	of Administration	Dose & Routes Comments
Indications The major indication for use of Isoproterenol at this time is limited to treatment of bradycardia that develops in the denervated transplanted heart- *- IF the drug should ever be used at all . . .* (AHA Text- Pg 1-32; 8-6).	**IV Infusion**- Mix **1mg** in **250 ml** of D5W- and begin drip @ **30 drops/ min (=2 µg/min)**. Titrate infusion to clinical effect (but do *not* exceed 10 µg/min].	Isoproterenol has become a *deemphasized drug*. It is *contraindicated* for treatment of asystole, EMD and V Fib because it increases myocardial oxygen consumption- and its pure beta-adrenergic effect results in vasodilatation (which *lowers* aortic diastolic pressure and therefore *reduces* coronary flow]). At low doses (i.e., <10 µg/min], Isoproterenol may provide pure chronotropic support to *selected* bradycardic pts who are not hypotensive. *The drug should not be used at higher doses.* At the present time, Epinephrine and/or Dopamine are generally preferred to Isoproterenol for use as "pressor agents".